Joy of Health

A Spiritual Concept of Integration and the Practicalities of Living

By ***Kathy Oddenino, RN***

Second Edition

The material in this book is provided for enlightenment only. Any action taken based upon the contents of this book is the sole responsibility of the reader.

Printed in the United States of America
ISBN 978-0-923081-08-9

First Edition published 1989

Requests for information or permission to make copies of any part of this work may be addressed to:
Joy Publications
241 Log Barn Acres Road, Pittsboro, NC 27312
919 545 9937

Edited by Margaret Martin
Cover and text design by Anita Crouch

DEDICATION

This book is dedicated to my parents Clarence M. Heskett, Emily L. Heskett, and my older sister Jane Heskett Jezek who I feel taught me more than any of the colleges that I attended. My parents taught me the value of living from a pure Nature, and how to never wait for someone else to do something for you, but learn to do everything in life for yourself. My sister Jane was my best friend and we lived as fellow explorers of Nature, life, and living. In learning to be my own person through their influences, I have grown into the truth of supporting my physical, mental, and emotional health, which has provided me with a fabulous life and a long life. I have written this book to help other people understand that we are one with Nature and we are created from a pure Nature, which helps us to understand and appreciate the secrets of Nature as the eternal and internal chemical support of our health and happiness in our human body and in our human life, and which has provided me with happiness, health, and a long life. Eating from Nature means that we do not eat foods that have chemicals on them or added to them. I am eternally grateful for my family and my friends for their patience, their wisdom, and their love.

ACKNOWLEDGEMENTS

I have been extremely fortunate in my life to have many wonderful and dedicated friends who believe in the Spiritual Philosophy that I teach. It is some special few of these friends that have supported me in helping to publish my many books on Spiritual Philosophy. When something important occurs in your life, the Universe will provide if you let it. Intellectually, I understand this concept but sometimes for me I have been slow to respond. I understand the Universal Energy that each of us lives, but understanding is not always physical mastery. How can anyone ever show the proper respect and love for the support of other people?

This is the second printing of The Joy of Health. I have had many people tell me that this one book has changed their life completely. As a Registered Nurse, it has always been my goal to help people understand the pure joy of living a healthy life from the foods of Nature, which I learned from my parents while I lived on our farm as a child. Life can be a challenge when we find ourselves sick all of the time. Medications do not take the place of a healthy diet and a healthy lifestyle. Acknowledge yourself, your wisdom, and your understanding of your human body, and then make it your goal to live the purity of health, in what you think, breathe, drink, eat, and physically do as you live. You are in total charge of your own health and happiness. No one else can do it for you.

In October 1930 I was born "sick" in the small town of Salem, Illinois, which I will always call home. No one expected me to live from year to year as a child, but I have defied the odds of health that I started with, and now I am healthier than I have ever been in my life. After high school I enrolled in a nursing school program in Indianapolis, Indiana. After I graduated from nursing school, I moved to Washington, DC to work in a research position in Tuberculosis. We found the cure for TB in 1951 and it is still being used today. Later in my life I did research with the HLA and DNA through an NIH program.

My family and my friends are a great support system and I appreciate each of them. I want to acknowledge Anita Crouch, Margaret Martin, Lucy Eckroth, and all of the loyal individuals that have supported me in the publication of the second edition of Joy of Health.

Thank you, each and every one of you for being in my life.

Joy of Health
A Message to the Reader

The Joy of Health is the true birthright of every human being. We start creating our reality the moment we are born.

Within the covers of this book you will find a Spiritual perspective of life and living. It is offered as an image of what can be, in relationship to our health and happiness. If you want to understand, you will. If you read with a closed mind, you won't. The concepts are many times opposite to the belief system that we are living. Try not to judge, and stay open of mind and heart as you read. We have created our own personal reality of disease as a nation and as a world, and now is the time for us to change how we believe, think, and act because we deserve to live a healthy life.

It is comforting to know that we can always change, and that is precisely what we must do if we want to live in health. This message is a "how to" commentary for being healthy in body, mind, and Spirit. It is presented lovingly and with common-sense wisdom. Understanding these concepts will give each of you the hope, love, and happiness that you may have considered impossible to find in your life. It is not easy for us to accept that we create our own reality in our physical body, mind, emotions, and in the world by the everyday thoughts that flash through our minds, and the everyday actions that result from these thoughts. Think about your life as you read. Try to relate the examples to your own life as you live it. *Do this without judgment, and with a sincere desire to understand You.* This book is an overview of the effect of the mind upon the body, but man (female or male) also has a Spirit that can never be separated from the mind and body. Therefore, the text approaches the human as a whole person and shows the integration of our physical life and our growth. Each commentary is considered essential to our human energy balance or it would not appear.

The subject matter in this book that relates to disease and health, represents the design of us as human beings. For our human design to be effective we must *believe in Spiritual Truth* and be committed to the truth of our eternal Energy. If you cannot believe in these truths, follow your present beliefs until you have the power to change your physical belief system. Attempting to follow Spiritual guidance when you deny personal responsibility will not be effective. For those who believe, healing will require a commitment to change. Change is the miracle of our human energy.

All of us have created dis-ease, disease, and dramas for ourselves sometime in our physical life; that is part of being human. When we can get out of our own way and stop resisting change, we can create vibrant health and joy just as easily. If it is your choice to follow the health regimen of the *Joy of Health,* you must be responsible for your own choice. I cannot be personally responsible for the choices you make. The Joy of Health requires your total commitment to the integrated balance of your body, mind, and Spirit Energy. No one has the power to change you, but you. If you choose to believe and seek an integrated balance in your life, you will find it.

Be in peace and joy,

Kathy Oddenino, RN

Commentaries

Introduction

A Spiritual concept of the integration of energy and its influences on our physical growth and our physical life

Man and Medicine *pg 1*

History of medicine... Hippocrates... Hohenheim... Wallace Yater... John Langley. Man and Nature... Balance of Nature... Bridge between the old and the new... Change as growth. As medicine has progressed through the ages, we have lost our consideration of Nature as the healer of our body and mind... Excesses and Deficiencies are the Promoters of Disease... Eternal Cycles of life and learning have been pushed aside in deference to money and fame

« Eternal Cycles of Life and Learning *pg 21*

The Bridge of Body and Mind *pg 23*

The human being is a creation of Spirit as energy and matter... Purpose of creation... Focus of healing both beliefs and the body. Possible life span on Earth... Changing of lifestyle... Definition of good health... Beliefs and health... Excesses and deficiencies...Alkaline-acid balance and disease

and his relationship to Nature… Man and his Soul and Spirit… Looking within, being open to the true perception of Self. Look at your world… Our creation of self and our Earth reality… Soul evolution and material gain… Ending the cycle of development… Aware souls are excited to be entering a new cycle of life

Second Cycle of Life *pg 175*

Beginning the cycle of Awareness, the second season… Imagine three equal circles… Soul memory… The Dual Soul is designing a program to Clean House … Effects of the Sun and Moon on the mind of man… The root cause of all fear within us… Soul cultures… Group cultures on Earth… Earth as a school, a learning center with many classrooms… Life as a classroom… Choice… Accepting responsibility for self, opening to Spiritual awareness… Learn about self… Choose wisely… the Law of Compensation, Balance… Free will… Our perception creates our reality… the power of experience and understanding what we gain from our experiences of life… Understanding the relationship of right or wrong to the issue of judgment, as dictated by time… the illusion of time, the reality of timelessness, synchronicity… Life is a choice, caring for our physical self which is subject to the Laws of Physical Matter… developing awareness is the most exciting, creative gift we can give ourselves

disease… Acts of love… AIDS… CANCER… PSORIASIS… ARTHRITIS… HEART-VASCULAR DISEASE… Disease in general… Causes and cures. All diseases can be cured… We are what we eat… Use it or lose it!

Our Responsibility *pg 313*

Fresh Air, Pure Water, Foods of Nature

Us and Our health… Air, water, and food… Accepting responsibility for health… Processed foods, fast-foods and our health… Compromising cellular viability… "Garbage In, Garbage Out"…Why have less than "perfect sex"?.. True teachers are also leaders

Addictions *pg 327*

Addiction – the opposite of freedom… Resisting change… Attachments… Purpose-survival… Addictions and Allergies… Who are we hiding from?… The belief system… Life is the ultimate in a beautiful chain… True Value… Spirit is Energy, We are Energy… Be honest… Drugs… Alcohol… Smoking… Loving yourself… Cure for addiction

Healing *pg 349*

Lessons in Will, Intent, and Healing

Our Spiritual Prospectus is designed with great care… Healing is an internal process… The human as healer… The energy of love… Validation of self… Miracle healings…There is no true death of energy… Death and dying… Spirit participation… Participants in the drama… Trilocular energy… Action and reaction.

Love *pg 367*

Emotions and their opposites… Essence of Spirit self… True emotional health is Spiritual growth… Everything has its purpose… Perfection in human beings… Love is freedom… Ego and the Spirit self… Old Souls… Love on Earth

Relationships *pg 391*

Soul lessons and JOY… Relationships- Casual… Families… Friends… Business… Lovers… Homosexuality… Solitary state… Karma (many people will experience but fail to learn)… "Laundry" day… Spiritual prospectus… Unconditional love

Marriage *pg 409*

Symbolic need… Male-Female roles… New Souls and old Souls… Marriage as a growth experience… Homosexual – Heterosexual marriage… Partnerships… Unconditional love… Abusive marriages… Mirror of self…

« Metaphysical Teachings, Levels of our invisible energy pg 426

The Spirit Self *pg 427*

Us and our relationship to Spirit… Nothing on Earth is an accident… Living is our lesson… Nature, Spirit and Human… Looking within… Perfect balance… The Spirit of Being… The Joy of Health

« Trinities of Ethical Values pg 438

INTRODUCTION

There is a very human purpose to my "madness." I love the energy of matter. I enjoy the energy of my Spirit Consciousness that I use in my physical life. I am a normal, functioning member of society that has lived with a different level of awareness than some of you. The different level of awareness that I have enjoyed was chosen as a prerequisite to the completion of my life purpose. The completion of my life purpose is also a completion of my Soul purpose, which is to learn the true Spirit energy of the nervous system and share it with others.

At this point in my Soul evolution, I am truly dedicated to the advancement of all Souls on Earth. In this respect, I share Soul energy with many of you. I am not different than you even though I may be, on a conscious level, more aware than some of you. I am and always have been well grounded in my physical reality. I chose this need for grounding and worked on its development for many years of my life. This established grounding has provided me with the comfort zone which I felt would be necessary for me to begin this work.

My Spirit does not have the ability to make me do something that I do not fully understand. With this first book we have chosen to reveal how the Soul and Spirit (mind, emotions, and senses) as energy works with the physical body on Earth. Our Souls are integrated and our writing is integrated. Because of this my Soul involves itself with my Spirit in experiencing the information that I share. My involvement is essential to the message I am communicating. We must feel comfortable with the work that we are doing. We work as one, we are one, but we are also separate. That is how we, as Souls, exist in the concept of our relationship to Spirit. We are energy as the essence of Spirit, and we are matter as our human design on Earth.

I came to this incarnation for a purpose and I have maintained that purpose. That doesn't mean that life has been easy or without challenges. My life has truly been a life of challenging experiences. But my lessons are mine and I face them with Spirit and an openness to further Soul evolution. I have lived my life with a consciousness of my Spirit energy and Spirit guides. They have not been there to make decisions for me but to support me in my own growth as it developed from my own needs. There have been in my life consistent guides and an array of guides, which have come and gone as my Soul has evolved. All Souls on Earth have similar guides to guide them through the art of living on Earth, but few are open to their presence.

I chose a difficult path of opposites to allow my vision to be complete. My Soul name is JOY and I requested that my Soul name follow me in this incarnation, although I have not been known as Joy. The very act of having JOY present in this reality has given me JOY. My Soul has incarnated many times and has run the gamut, so to speak, from Saint to sinner. As with many souls, my talents are many more than I have chosen to use. I have chosen to be a teacher of healing in this life for the evolution of Souls on Earth. I have maintained that focus even when faced with the temptation of change and wealth.

Maintaining the focus of nursing, with a Soul awareness of healing, has presented many instances when I could have chosen to heal the patient with Spiritual wisdom when the physician failed in scientific wisdom. Had I bent to this temptation, I would have lost my focus for our work from the external interference of the physical world. I have chosen to maintain my energy focus and separate the physical reality that I enjoy from the Spiritual reality. It was necessary for me to come to Earth many thousands of times before the dawning of this time period. Being a Spiritual conduit made me uncomfortable and I chose to train vigorously in this lifetime until I could create a comfort zone from which to work. My comfort zone was not created from money or material possessions but from the joining of Souls that love and support me in what I need to do. These Souls that have traveled through the energy systems together and with me are my comfort zone.

The capability for healing and teaching has always been there as a Soul memory for me and has been exercised to a degree. Still, I have manifested amazing resistance to my final Soul revelation. My decision to train for this revelation from the awareness level of nursing was determined before my decision to incarnate. Many of my lifetimes have been spent in the field of medicine and healing so the choice of nursing was appropriate. It was also significant from the relationship of opposites, and as such, it has provided the perfect classroom for viewing the opposites of humanity as well as the opposite concepts of cause and effect in health versus disease.

My Spirit Consciousness has evolved on Earth and has transcended to another plane where my own evolution continues. We are each part of the same Soul. We have other levels of Souls that are part of us. At this time in my life we are in communication on a Higher Spirit Level. Other Spirit guides on the level of the sixth plane interact with our energy. Their Spirit names are Socrates and Joy. These energies could be called an Oversoul. We are all one Soul in the Spirit world. When we reach our total evolution we become light and can be all places at once. There is much work on many planes before we can hope to evolve to that level. But, as in other things, the fun is also found in the doing. We will cover the subject of Soul evolution another time. The human Spirit and the infinite evolution of the Soul is in itself another book. As a Soul I have evolved through thousands of incarnations and some of these incarnations can be found documented in writings of our world today. Even in this respect, I am not different. That comment could be made by every person. Each Soul travels through the same experiences to learn, as their need to deal with that issue becomes apparent to the eternal Soul and Spirit.

In this book we are dealing with the body as physical matter and the inter-relationship of the body and mind. We cannot separate the Spirit, as we are born as an integrated energy SELF living in matter. Our Spirit energy is our motivation to life and living. But the important place for us to begin in understanding SELF is in the part of self that we relate to in this moment of our physical existence. The physical human is physical matter that is controlled by our mind. Putting the physical SELF in perspective as an integrated part of Earth is our goal for this book.

We are dealing with health and the joy that is found in understanding what health truly means to us on Earth. Health is not simply one issue but many issues with individual impact on the three parts of our human body. It is impossible to maintain health of one integral as the body, mind, and Spirit without maintaining health of the other two. As human beings we are energy and matter that is controlled and expanded through the design of our internal nervous system that begins with our brain as consciousness.

The energy waves are interwoven and inseparable. Our strength comes from three separate energy sources – the Infinite Spirit Energy (Spirit), the Universal Energy (Soul – emotions and mind), and the Earth Energy (body). We are trilocular beings moving with centripetal force as we seek the balance of self on Earth. Incarnation on Earth requires a grounding on Earth (human body) from which to function as an energy rhythm of Nature. When we upset that rhythm by denial of our physical body then we cease to be on Earth. In our human terms, our body experiences a physical death. Denial of our body can be manifested through any of the three integrates.

If a mother is to give birth to twins there will be three integrates involved in the process. If the mother or either infant develops a problem, the two that are left in temporary good health are suddenly at risk. Therapeutic intervention can change that risk factor, but without it the problem can escalate. Intervention could mean that one or two of the integrates could be saved, and in life we can be saved for a long time with damage to one or more integrates, but the eventual outcome is evolutionary blockage. Blockage is to be avoided whenever possible. An *integrate* is a "soul" that is choosing a method of entry as an energy.

When the Soul becomes aware of a terminal blockage it usually decides to leave. It can manifest its leaving in many ways, from a normal death, self-inflicted death, tragic or traumatic death, or a disease-ridden death. The final decision has been made to leave and it is the Soul's choice of how that will be accomplished. Our goal is to help you evaluate your own health by raising your awareness level of the integration of body, mind, and Spirit which will help you live and prevent many challenges. As we think, we create the energy of our thoughts, which we reflect into our physical reality.

As human beings, we never lose the influence of the energy sources that surround us and course through us as a river through the Earth. These forces, as the energy of the nervous system, suffer the low and high tides of Nature which depend on the rhythm of the individual to the chemicals available in Nature. These rivers of energy control the body, mind and Spirit as they are part of the body, mind and Spirit as our design. Within each of us there is a trilogy of force energy. That energy IS the creation of us. The trilogy of force energy is our body, mind and Spirit. Other energies exist as consciousness energy forces. The influences of the consciousness energy forces which act as bridges of consciousness are discussed in my second book, *Bridges of Consciousness.*

This is not a technical book about health but rather a Spiritual concept of integration of the body, mind, and Spirit self and its influences on the practicality of living. The contents will not necessarily agree with scientific material or interpretation, but it is truth from a higher level of understanding. If you are ready for it, it will automatically read as truth to you. We are presenting this book "to the masses" as an overview for understanding healthy living. We have not approached any subject in depth, because our focus with this work is to trigger awareness within the human mind that we are energy first and physical matter on the second level. In later books we will explore many individual subjects more fully to help with the understanding of energy and matter as two levels of us.

There are no defined chapters in the *Joy of Health* because there are no possible separations in the true physical creation of the joy of health. We have simply chosen essential creations of living that we are speaking of in an integrated way. It is my intention to show you how each of these happenings of life impact on our health and joy in our daily life. Our creations are separate but integrated and they each influence the whole of life with a profound and creative impact. If we could separate them, we would have to call them body, mind and Spirit influences that function in an integrated way. Our physical health is created by our attitudes and beliefs, and all of these creations can be changed and newly created by our Spiritual awakening. I offer this explanation as an alternate definition of the joy of health.

My Spirit and I have had a continuous transmission for an infinite period. It is our plan, for the future, to maintain an endless written transmission that will be available to all. If the human Soul is ready to awaken, we will join with it to trigger that awareness within. If our awareness can be awakened, we can grow from the development cycle of life to the awareness cycle, to the understanding cycle and then we can learn to integrate all that we have learned. It is this fourth cycle of life, the cycle of integration, that brings peace and joy into our life.

Abraham Maslow understood this cycle, just as Carl Jung did, but neither could fully integrate it and explain it to the average person so that he could clearly understand. Rudolph Steiner was another person that understood. Steiner integrated the Spiritual understanding more completely than Maslow or Jung. Another researcher who looked at the body carefully, especially the entire nervous system, was John Newport Langley, an Englishman of great renown. These men were old Souls when they were attempting to explain the body, mind and Spirit. Today, they are older Souls and they live again on Earth. In more current times, Wallace Yater (1895-1976), a physician in Washington, DC, was a man who returned into this life with many lifetimes of memories about our human body and its health, which he lived in his role as a physician.

I mention these men that you may recognize, because I want each of you to know that what I am writing about is not new, nor has it been unrecognized by the human mind. Many people have understood these concepts, centuries before the ones that I have mentioned. It is unfortunate that we have lost sight today of how we were created. Within our dialogue is the truth of creation on all levels. It is my wish that we can prove to you the Joy of Health that is the true birthright of each and every human being.

MAN AND MEDICINE

Hippocrates was a Greek physician who lived approximately 5,000 years ago, in our time, before the birth of Jesus Christ. He has been honored by our world as the first physician to practice the Art of Medicine. Hippocrates did practice Medicine as an art. He is considered to be the Father of Medicine. It is truly an honor that this advanced Soul deserves. The Soul that was Hippocrates has lived hundreds of lives since the life when he was known as the Father of Medicine. He has continued to be in medicine for many of his physical lives. He has faced the same struggles that all physicians face when they want medicine to be an art but they must treat it as a science in our culture of today.

For many years, physicians took the "Hippocratic Oath" when they graduated from medical school. This oath has become part of the culture of medicine. Few physicians follow Hippocrates in practicing medicine as he practiced medicine as an art of Nature. The Nature in medicine has been misplaced by the chemicals in medicine. Hippocrates treated the human being in relationship to the rhythm of Nature, by using the elements of Nature.

Understanding the relationship of man to Nature was the most significant art that Hippocrates used. He understood the relationship between the rhythm of the body to the rhythm of the Earth. This relationship was the basis of all his medical treatments. Hippocrates had an innate sense of knowing and understanding the consciousness streams that attach the human body to the body of Earth. It was in this natural rhythm that he was comfortable and at peace. In the mind of Hippocrates, the human was one with Nature. He was another organism living from and with that natural rhythm of restoration and growth from the energy of Earth.

Hippocrates understood the elements of the Earth and he used them freely in restoring his patients to health. He did not consciously understand his closeness to Spirit during that lifetime. But the consciousness did not have to be present for him to function from his unconscious Spiritual energy. In this respect humans are all the same. We function every day from our unconscious Spiritual perspective. It is this unconsciousness of energy that reflects the Spiritual perspective that keeps us closer to the rhythm of Nature than we consciously realize.

Hippocrates understood the inter-relationship between the rhythm of the body and the rhythm of the Earth. He knew that within the fruits of the Earth were the cures for human ills. He knew that we, too, are organisms of the Earth, just as every other organism is a product of the Earth. There are no new organisms on Earth, but their virulence has changed. All that is, has been. But organisms can be made more virulent with man-made chemicals. The imbalance on Earth gives dormant germs strength and purpose.

Hippocrates understood that the human is the most highly evolved of Earth's organisms. He knew that physical evolution required us to live from the living plants of Earth, just as less evolved organisms live from other less evolved organisms. He understood that attunement to Nature was the healthy way for us to live. Laws of Nature control the life of Earth. Survival of the fittest is a Law of Nature. This law does not refer only to human fitness but also to the fitness of all organisms. The strongest organism is the natural survivor. When an organism becomes stronger than the human being, it is an indication of imbalance within the human body.

In the line of evolution we are the strongest organism when we abide by the Laws of Nature. When we fail to abide by the Laws of Nature we lower our natural resistance to Nature's organisms. Lowering the resistance of the body makes the human body more susceptible to the increased growth of organisms. We are sending the organisms that are compatible with us in strength, a silent message of relinquishment. We are saying in the language of organisms, "It is your turn to be strong." The growth of these parasitic organisms within our human body will create disease, and most of us will not understand that we have allowed this excess growth when it happens.

The Laws of Nature are consistently in operation on Earth. Failure to maintain the necessary balance of

Nature is one issue in our human health today. We have attempted to remove ourselves from the rhythm of Nature. We have turned to science and the discoveries of science. We have begun to believe that we cannot survive without the discoveries of science. Our science has given us time to recover our balance. Science does not cure, it "fixes," or it "treats," but it can also kill. There is great humor in our phrase, "the practice of medicine" for it is indeed practice, and hopefully we will all in time learn how to use Nature as our medicine of choice.

Science is, by definition, the study of natural phenomena. The most effective of the scientific studies are those that study human experience. We need to study the experience of health, not disease. The most useful study for all humans is studying the effects of the rhythm of Nature and its personal effect on us. In our present culture, we fail to appreciate the inter-relationship between our body and the living Earth. Earth is there to provide us with the elements we need to remain healthy and happy as a human being. The Nervous System functions from these chemicals of Nature. Without a nervous system where would we be today? Crawling on our belly, for sure.

Disease within the body is by nature a chemical imbalance within our body and mind. The disease itself is not important. The balance and maintaining the balance is the prevention and the cure for the disease. We are not aware of the impact of the interference which science creates within this natural rhythm that exists between us and the Earth that supports our life. Hippocrates was an advocate of remaining close to the Earth. He used the elements of the Earth to treat diseases. Air and water therapy, nutritional therapy and herbal therapy were the medicines he relied upon. These natural elements restore the rhythm of human beings with the Earth, from which we find our essential and vital source of energy.

The scientific change in the practice of medicine occurred in our world around 1500 AD. This change was the result of a physician by the name of Phillip von Hohenheim, who later took the name Paracelsus. Hohenheim was born in Switzerland in 1493, and has been described as a Renaissance physician, botanist, alchemist, astrologer, and general occultist. (He is said to have died at age 48 of "natural causes.") He was the first of Earth's physicians to practice medicine as a science. Hohenheim began the use of deadly drugs to treat diseases. His drugs were sometimes so deadly that the patient died as a result of the cure. The use of drugs has increased through the years of advancing science and drugs have increased to our benefit and detriment.

The benefits of the scientific advances are many. They allow all of us the privilege of awareness of health versus disease, as a Soul lesson. The physician can fix or treat some problems which will give us the time to heal ourselves. Let us use an example: Take a forty-five-year-old man who lives a life of stress and anger. He works sixteen hours a day. He takes no time off to have fun. He doesn't understand the words "joy" and "happiness." Since he works so hard and so consistently, he never sees his family. Now his marriage is "on the rocks." One day our hard-working man begins to have severe pain in his heart. He is admitted to the hospital and he is treated. He lives to go home.

At this point our man has reached a cross-roads in his life. He now has a choice to make. Is he going to continue the work schedule and continue the stress, as the imbalance that he is presenting to his mind and body? Or is he going to work less, play more and learn to enjoy his family and his life? Our man has been presented with a choice. Science gave him the opportunity, by saving his life, to have the time for a choice. These are the benefits of the science of medicine. Every human is given an opportunity to change in his physical lives. If our man does not change he will continue to be presented with more opportunities to die, until finally, medicine cannot keep him alive any longer.

Once we can understand that options are important we can seriously consider our options as valid to our physical experience. The benefit of the medical treatment creates the opportunity for us to change. The opportunity for change is what medicine can provide. Only this man can change the condition of his heart. Heart problems are symbolic of the need for love. When we are not eating right, we do not love ourselves. Each of us is responsible for balancing our work, our life, our behaviors, our thinking and what we eat and drink. This man is responsible for his choice of change. Each of us is also responsible for giving and receiving love in our life.

The detriment of the science of medicine is found in the perception that physicians can heal all disease. Medicine is seen by many people as being totally responsible for their overall health. This is a fallacy that we have allowed ourselves to live with as a false sense of security in our total reliance on medical treatment as a "quick fix." Medical treatment does not remove the responsibility of each and every human being to take care of self. Science can treat and it can sometimes create a temporary "cure," but we are always responsible for the overall change in our lifestyle that will create the lasting cure. It is the responsibility of each and every individual to create the balance in living that will create good health. This can be accomplished by restoring the natural balance of the human body through Nature. Today's many medicines place the body in an extreme state of imbalance if great caution is not used.

All of humankind is involved in learning the lesson of physical balance. Teaching ourselves the balance of the physical chemicals within our human body is a lesson that is being learned on Earth but, to date, it has not been taught through medicine. Lessons are taught on Earth by the truth in the experience of opposites. As we learn, we have the power of change to work with. Seeing what does and what does not work opens the awareness levels of the human mind. Understanding the lesson of opposites can only be accomplished when each person is ready to see the reality of the physical experience. Disease is a lesson of opposites. Health is the opposite of disease. We must understand chemical imbalance as the root cause of the disease within our life, to cure the disease within our body.

Now it is becoming obvious in our world that our reliance on drugs and chemicals is producing an economic burden of disease in all humans. The diseases escalate as the drugs escalate. The further from Nature's balance that we go, the more the body is forced into a state of chemical imbalance. There is a Law of Physical Matter and a Law of Energy that dictate the viability of our cellular structure. Most of us refuse to look within ourselves and our life for the true cause of disease. We refuse to hear that rhythm of Nature that we are attuned to. Instead, we will place the responsibility for our disease on any distorted belief that we can imagine. We do not enjoy hearing that we create our own personal reality in life, including the diseases of the entire human race. When we cannot understand our relationship to Nature, how can we possibly understand our relationship to disease?

Medicine has created our thinking through many years of the evolution of Earth's time. What started out to be treatment as an art has now become treatment by medicine. Medicine has accepted the responsibility to cure by scientific knowledge and partially ignore Nature. We have learned to deny the responsibility of healing self and given the responsibility of healing to the medical community and to drugs. Today we look to science to cure all ills rather than all humans working to balance our body and mind with Nature. Chemicals that are foreign to our body cannot and will not support the health of our human chemical design.

Excesses and Deficiencies are the Promoters of Disease.

Few people really stop and ask themselves, "What can I do to help myself?" When anything becomes excessive it is by nature unbalanced, which includes any addiction to another person to heal us, or for drugs to heal us. Excesses and deficiencies are the promoters of disease. Excesses and deficiencies are the immediate reaction to the imbalance, the root cause of which is within the mind. The current thought of the average person, that he must be restored to health by the intervention of science, is a failure to accept personal responsibility for his own personal and individual relationship to Nature. The scientific dependency of society has the force of materialism supporting its continual growth. The commercialization of the Art of Medicine is the direct cause of our diseases of senility. They need not be, if the balance of Nature within us is honored. These diseases of senility are a destructive force in our society. There is the moral destruction of impending senility for each of us and the economic destruction of our financial security. This financial security affects not only the individual person in our society but it affects our entire culture through the world of our government.

The practice of medicine as a materialistic science leads to a gross imbalance in the human body and our societal system. Dependency practice promotes a gross imbalance within our Soul growth process. It encourages the Soul to leave the physical body before the completion of the Earth lesson. The lesson of the Dual Soul becomes overwhelmed and frustrated with the denial of the lesson of Nature and its necessary balance, as we forego personal responsibility for dependency on drugs.

The first lesson of Earth is learning to maintain the balance of the rhythms between us and Nature. It is learning to balance the physical, at all times. This is survival of the fittest, in the sense of the physical body on Earth. When we promote imbalance, we are promoting disease. Any excess or deficiency in life is a creation or promotion of disease. We cannot be removed from the energy and balance of Nature and live with Joy. Science has learned to maintain the function of physical matter artificially for a period of time. The opposite of living and life then becomes an issue of defining death.

Today, the world of medicine needs to find its balance. The knowledge is greater in the scientific arena than it has ever been since the last great change occurred on Earth. The last dramatic change that occurred on Earth happened in the time that we refer to as Atlantis.

Change will always occur on Earth when our values are focused on material cravings. Human evolution must be focused within the mind and body, not without. When the focus becomes external, it creates an imbalance within the internal mind, body and evolving Soul of the human being. We are on Earth to learn our own perfection. Now we can learn to integrate the best of the art with the best of science. Now we have evolved enough that we must learn to bridge that gap, to ensure our survival within the seasons of life on Earth.

The Scientific diagnosis of physical problems must be integrated with the understanding of the lesson the individual has planned to learn. Understanding the lesson will allow us to participate in the treatment therapy that will best restore the natural rhythm of the body and Dual Soul mind. Learning the coordination of the mind and body is an art that promotes growth of the Dual Soul and Spirit Consciousness. Our Scientific focus of chemical therapy is a detriment to the viability of the human cellular design and function. We are capable, with guidance, of self-healing and prevention of disease.

Dis-ease and disease are an avoidance response of the mind within the human body. When you are happy, don't you feel good? Be conscious in your daily living of exactly what moments give you joy and happiness. Avoidance is promoted by the mind through the excesses and deficiencies of our physical life. We create excesses and deficiencies when we cannot openly face some reality of our creation of everyday life. Avoidance has never solved any problem in our evolution and it will not solve problems today.

Let us use an example: Let's observe a man who is living what is considered a good life. He has everything that money can buy. He has freedom to travel. He has a good job. He is intelligent, handsome and charming. But our man has an excessive behavior that he has created. He is an alcoholic. Our man has everything from the standpoint of the material and the intellectual. He has a good body. He has a good mind. What he hasn't yet developed in his world is his Soul and Spirit. What is the Soul and Spirit of our world? The manifestation of the Spirit in the physical world is the love that comes from the heart of us. This is not love of the material life. This is love as an emotion that is given and received from the heart. This is the love of self and thy neighbor that is the essence of the Love of Spirit.

Denial of the need to openly examine a relationship, whether this is between two individuals, a work situation, a financial situation or whatever drama of life, will result in dis-ease. Dis-ease can escalate into disease of the body and mind if the pattern is not changed. If the individual cannot openly confront what is bothering him, the body will respond with a delaying tactic. It will become diseased. The excess of alcohol can and will destroy the viability of the cellular structure. Our man is promoting or creating disease as a way of death, and he is being supported in his decision by his Dual Soul and Spirit Consciousness. He has chosen a course of self-destruction and he is fully aware of the choice that he has made internally if not consciously.

Encouraging ourselves to maintain the balance of Nature through AIR, WATER, and FOODS from the EARTH will help with the annoyances of physical imbalance. It is the "worried well" who have dis-ease. They are in such a confused state of imbalance that their body is telling them, on a subconscious level, to seek balance. Seeking medical treatment by a physician may add to this imbalance if the physician is practicing from the scientific concept of health. Not only might the physician give drugs willingly, but if he withholds chemical treatment the patient may feel offended and abused. As the human race, we need to become aware of the effects of drugs and chemicals within the chemical human body.

Drugs present the immediate problem of compounding our already existing imbalance. It is only our belief system that makes us feel that chemical treatment is essential because emotionally we feel ill. It is not the physical complaint that makes it essential. The patient and the physician would both be more balanced, if the physician could communicate and the patient could hear and accept advice for balancing the body naturally. The ability to balance the body and mind naturally, rather than using a chemical substitute, is an internal and external process for us. Every person should understand that we have the ability to heal ourselves from cancer as well as other diseases. *The body has its own powers of healing which are not currently being used by the masses.*

Scientific treatment is often administered innocently and received innocently, because neither the patient nor the physician is truly in tune with Nature. The Hippocratic Oath that was taken by physicians says: "I swear…to heal…according to my ability and judgment," yet in today's world, the judgment and ability of the physician is frequently not accepted by the patient. It is common to have as many opinions on a disease as we have physicians involved. This promotes distrust within the patient. Radical procedures are common and generally unnecessary, if the patient will accept the responsibility to change his or her life. If the patient has chosen the lesson of physical death, all measures will be unsuccessful. If the patient has chosen the disease for awareness, nothing more will be necessary to effect a cure.

Hippocrates understood Nature and responded unconsciously in a period of evolution when balance was crucial to his teaching. He wanted to do no harm to man by deed or word. He truly helped the person to help himself. This was a creative approach in a time when that was essentially the only approach. This approach created the *Art of Medical Care* and it deserves the greatest honor, because it has saved many lives.

Many physicians today are old Souls. This is not the first time they have accepted the responsibility for helping us to help ourselves. Physicians who base all their treatment on the scientific approach rather than the artistic approach are Souls from a more recent creation. In life the level of Souls will seek each other. A Soul with inner knowing will not be comfortable with the scientific approach. A Soul that has evolved in the scientific level will not feel comfortable with a holistic approach. None of life is right or wrong. It is only the level of the Soul, and it is perfect for the lesson the Soul is striving to understand.

We have evolved to a much greater degree today than the Soul of Hippocrates experienced during the incarnation when he was known as Hippocrates the physician. Evolution is life and life is evolution. We continue to create one life after the other in our repetitious learning process of being human. We do not get to stop our evolution and go to live with Spirit, because that is not the way that we were designed as a constantly evolving energy. The Human is evolving in the development, awareness, understanding and integration that we are experiencing in our multiple lives. Throughout time we have developed our Ethical Values that are now helping us to grow, change, and evolve into a higher level of evolving energy.

Life is the normal change of "constant growth" for our internal energy fields. Without the willingness to change, we cannot grow. At this time in our evolution on Earth, it is time for another revolutionary change in our awareness of our relationship to the Earth, to the Universe and to Spirit energy as the creator of our energy pattern and design. Our intellectual change of beginning to understand the energy of us as human beings has the capability of elevating us out of the restrictions of the "physical" into the freedom of the "Spiritual" while we continue living an Earth life. We are creating this growth change to balance the thinking mind and loving emotions of our human Soul. When this change is called *evolution* it has some merit, but when it is called *revolutionary* change, it gives our multiple lives a design and a purpose that we may not appreciate without a better understanding of ourselves and our human design as an eternal energy being.

Through the ages of growth in the human design, we have evolved the science of medicine as we saw the need presented. Our focus has been away from the laws of Nature and closer to the realm of science. The advances of science are commendable and exciting, but the past and the present must be used as integrated concepts. We cannot be cured by science. Curing is an internal process that begins within our mind. Remember that the disease was created for the experience. The disease will remain until the awareness has been developed that can allow the Soul to understand the lesson of the disease.

The symbolism that Spirit created for us in the Garden of Eden spoke to our balance in all aspects of our BEING. When we choose to live from "the tree of knowledge" we will know guilt, greed, sorrow and pain.

The "tree of knowledge" is symbolic of the loss of balance with Nature that we are now experiencing on Earth. It is all-inclusive of the relationship of man and Nature. Spirit in its wisdom and awareness of human Soul evolution was telling us that we must always seek our balance within Nature, no matter what else we have learned or may be exposed to. This is why it is vitally important for us to eat food, drink water, and breathe air that has not been contaminated with any form of chemical. Our chemicals are causing disease. Spirit designed us with a need for the physical balance of the chemicals from a pure Nature within every cell within our human body, as a necessary action to balance our ego.

In the "knowledge" of the science of medicine, the need for balancing the body with the elements of Nature has been essentially lost. The imbalance in the elements is recognized and valued, but the way of Nature's balance is ignored by many. The awareness of the need for balance is seen and evaluated with a scientific perception rather than the perception of us as a part of Nature. We attempt to balance the imbalance with chemicals which in turn create their own imbalance. The ability of today's physician to bridge the gap between the art of medicine and the science of medicine is more real than it has ever been. The true Soul physician of today, who was motivated to enter the art of healing because of a Soul purpose to serve humankind, knows that something is truly missing in the art of medicine. True physicians understand on a Soul level that in order to live with joy and health, we must accept the responsibility of self and be committed to balancing ourselves with Nature. True healers will always be in demand in the world we live in because internally we object to the way medicine is practiced as a means to sell pills. Healers will be in demand not to prescribe the chemicals that are man's creations, but to guide us in our need to learn the ability to create a perfect balance within us which will promote excellent health and happiness. Physicians do not heal with drugs. The belief of the patient in the drugs allows temporary healing to occur, just as being in the presence of some physicians can heal some people.

The value of the physician is in the awareness and understanding that he has of the experience of disease. We are healed by our own internal understanding that we are not alone and in imminent danger of physical death. If we do not want to be healed, we will not be healed, despite the treatment that is administered by a physician. True healing happens when we understand that disease does not serve us anymore. Knowing that we will no longer use disease to avoid the issues of life, the love of self that we are all striving to access gives us the ability to recognize what we are doing and to heal our own body and mind. Accepting the responsibility for the balance of self will be the natural result of this understanding.

Dis-ease may be present for years before it will be manifested in the physical degeneration of some part of the human body. Dis-ease is an action of the mind and the reaction is found in various diseases of the physical. Anyone who feels that he is a paragon of physical health needs to be certain that he is living with inner peace and joy or disease will happen suddenly in his life. Bridging the gap in the world of medicine is the art involved in the practice of medicine today. It is not easy for a physician to be different in a scientific world. Being different in a scientific world creates distrust among our peers. This distrust is the result of judgment. Judgment creates categories of right and wrong as well as a huge amount of fear. There is no right and wrong. Life is lived to learn and it is only our perception that allows right and wrong to become tools of judgment.

Science looks at numbers and considers that the numbers that are found are the ultimate truth, which is considered proof of a theory. But it seeks proof through the negatives of medicine, rather than the positives. Within the true healings we can find the balance for ourselves. It is through looking at the experience of these healings that we will be aware of the conscious creation of health. Using the elements of Nature in healing would be a positive step for the physician of today. This is not to create a new world of excesses, but rather to balance the chemicals in the human cells. The elements of Nature that should be used are the air, the water and the first generation of foods of the Earth. Return to the natural. Forget man-made chemicals, processed food, and drugs. Become your own physician as you learn to eat the proper foods, drink the purest water that you can find, and use no chemicals in your home to keep yourself healthy and happy.

Be in tune with the energies of Earth that strengthen and protect the physical self. Learn that love is a healing energy. Begin by loving the self that you are. Show your appreciation of self by caring for the physical self. Tuning your energies with those of Nature will keep you healthy and happy in this life on Earth. Be aware of your surroundings. Awareness and understanding of our relationship to the living Earth and the energy that is there for us when we choose to use it will change our life on Earth. We will also change our relationship to living as a human being. Accept the responsibility to be all that you can be, physically and mentally. Give up your excesses and you will cure your deficiencies.

Use medicine sparingly. Use physicians to understand the disease which you have created. Understanding the disease will allow you to discern the root cause. Each and every disease is symbolic of an excess emotion or a lack of an emotion within us, which will always be aggravated by any excess in chemical consumption. Cure the problem of the mind and you will create a new body. We create the body that we live in through the direct use of the beliefs of our mind. Understanding that love is the elixir of health will give us permission to love and to be loved from the heart and Soul of self. Love will restore our JOY in our HEALTH and we will reap what we sow in the happiness and joy of living.

Eternal Cycles of Life and Learning

Know Thyself –
Spirit Consciousness – Dual Soul, Physical Body

Each life is an energy of expansion.

We are energy and we are matter.

Physical Body as our creation of our own energy reality.

Who we are as human beings

What we know

What we live

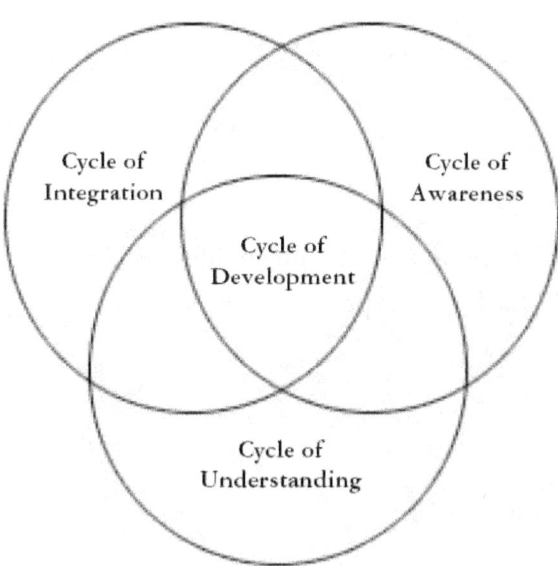

3 Dimensional View

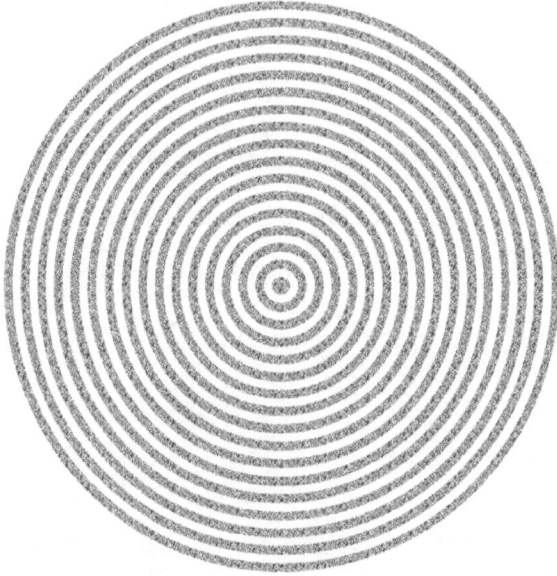

Development of human life from the Universal System. Each cycle represents our human evolution.

THE BRIDGE OF BODY AND MIND

The human is a creation of Spirit. We are created in Spirit's image as energy, and in Earth's image as matter. This does not necessarily mean that we look like Spirit, but we are made in the energy and matter as Spirit is thought to be made. We are body, mind, and Spirit. The energy of us bridges the physical matter of us and makes us human. Nothing new exists upon the Earth. It has all been before and will all be again. We are a continual recreation from the chemicals of Nature, Earth, and the Universe. Knowledge is a continued relearning and relating. There is nothing new to the human mind, only the details change and grow within our thinking mind. The information in this book is not new. We all know and understand the information on a Soul level. It has been written before and it will be written again.

Today it is necessary to bring this memory back again into the light of awareness because we have forgotten the rhythm of our being and the true source of that rhythm as our internal energy that is relating to the energy of Earth. In the earlier Soul cultures on Earth, growth concentration created our destruction and destruction of the society that we had established on Earth. Without awareness and understanding this destruction was as it had to BE and as it could BE again. It is very important for us as a human species to open our mind to the reality of eternal life on Earth. We have much to learn here and we will not leave planet Earth as our home until we complete our mission of learning.

Spirit does not let us forget our balance for long periods of time. To do that would not contribute to the true purpose of life on Earth, which is the evolution of the Dual Soul and Spirit Energy. The Soul cannot grow with a singular concentration of intent. We are a trilogy of Being. Between each of the parts there is a bridge that influences the function of the other part. As a closely structured unit, the whole is affected by each part and each part is affected by the whole. We cannot expand in only one part and protect the viability of the whole. Once we learn that we are energy and the Universe is energy we begin to see that we are intensely related to the Universe, Earth, Nature, and all life on Earth.

The human physical body is the expendable part of us. Our body is designed as the temple of the Spirit and Soul on Earth. It will return to dust as it came from dust. Our mind is a Universal Energy. All of the knowledge of the Universe is there when we learn to capture it within our consciousness memory. The Spirit energy is the eternal part of us. The Spirit of us is the image of Spirit, the Spirit self within us. The Spirit of us is the part of us that lives eternally as energy. Spirit designed us as one integrated unit with each part dependent upon the other part. It is the Spirit energy of us that is living as a means of learning how to be perfect as an expanding energy.

We were created for the purpose of Soul evolution. It is our intent as a human being to have all of the fragmented parts of SELF, which are now within us as body, mind, and Spirit, to grow, to evolve, and to meet the Spirit's own state of BEING. We are made in the Spirit image as energy. On Earth we have physical children and we expect them to grow to adulthood in our image. The reality of our physical life is a duplication of the reality of the Spirit world. As we grow, our Soul grows as an energy field. With the growth of the Soul on Earth, we learn to live in love rather than fear. On the higher levels of the Spiritual plane, there is no fear. There is only love among the Souls that have evolved enough to reach these unseen energy levels.

Health, as we know it on Earth, is primary to Soul evolution. Disease is a path of intense learning. Disease can also result in physical death and rebirth to continue the learning experience that was chosen as the life design. At this time on Earth there needs to be a blending of the old and the new. This is the perfect time for us to use the balance of Nature and blend it with the best of science, for an expanded awareness in the quality of living. At this time on Earth the concept of healing is out of balance with Nature. Healing has become captured by commercialism and fear. Soon there will be no healers willing to heal. Healing itself has taken the wrong focus.

Healing is not commercial. Healing is healing the energy within a physical body. We can heal more with Nature's food, air and water than we can heal with the medicine from science.

The fear that healers experience has changed medicine from an art to an adversarial science. Physicians cannot be healers when they are forced to protect themselves by being technicians. When society denies the freedom of the art of healing to the physician, we destroy the art and the joy of healing. We must learn to appreciate the healers that are on Earth. Society must give the privilege of healing back to the physician. Medicine has become a technical science because of the demands of medicine. Health care in general is not working as well for the health of everyone today, as it did when medicine was an intuitive and creative art. We are organic matter. We can only be restored with the organic matter of Nature, which is the air, water, and foods of Nature.

The elements of Nature allow us to live in a balanced rhythm of chemical energy. Removing the body from these energy rhythms, by the introduction of elements foreign to Nature, will create a negative energy. This negative energy will result in physical blockage and an imbalance of the integrated self. The current concept of medicine has provided some of us with more material possessions as a result of the increased commercialism of supply and demand of drugs. The present focus of medicine is not where true healing of the physical body is to be found on Earth. Medicine is not where the true balance of the body, mind and Spirit is to be found, and it is not where our health truly is capable of being supported.

Industrialization created commercialism which created materialism. Each was created for the survival of our belief system and business. None was truly created for the balance of our health, although we believe that they were. This creation has been offered to the Earth as our choice to compare the truth of health. In this choice is the image of opposites for the physical SELF. In the polarization of opposing forces, there is a lesson. We have the option, at this point on Earth, of choosing how we want to live, how long we want to live and what we want to learn in the process.

We can live well over one hundred years if that is our choice. It takes over one hundred years, in our time, to truly experience the four seasons of life. At this time in our culture, we seldom see the ending of the second season. Many Souls never experience the beginning or end fully. A few will choose two hundred and more years of life in our future time. Ways of healing can be used which will assure Souls of very long Earth lives. These long lives will be spent consciously working on their Soul evolution.

Understanding the role of the mind in health is the first step to healing. Understanding the care that one must offer the physical body is the second step. One cannot work without the other. The understanding of this bridge provides a mind, body coordination that is healthy and joyful from the moment of conscious awareness. With this awareness we can make a conscious choice of physical death, at any age. This understanding allows our body to be aware of the effect of all that it encounters. This awareness will allow us to consciously experience the positive and the negative effect of food, energy, and physical circumstance. Being aware gives us the choice of change. Many of us are now experiencing a restless, uneasy feeling that intrudes into our everyday lives. We cannot understand this feeling. This restlessness is the awakening of awareness which people are consciously suppressing. It is time for every human being to understand themselves at a more expansive level, which requires that all humans learn Spiritual Philosophy.

When awareness awakens, it normally demands that we change our lifestyle. Until this awareness is acceptable and desired by our total self as the body, mind and Spirit, that part of the mind that is controlled by the intellect and ego will continue to deny its existence. Along with this restless, uneasy feeling we will notice that we want more time away from the noise and clamor of daily survival. We will want to be alone or in peaceful company. There will be a gradual denial of fear and an embracement of love. Acquaintances of different ethical standards will dissolve from our reality and we will seek those of like energy vibrations. The Soul purpose of every Soul is learning, through living the experiences necessary for Soul evolution.

Learning comes in many forms. The ultimate in learning is the awareness of the JOY in BEING. In order to feel JOY IN BEING we must start with learning to live the JOY OF HEALTH, which is a lesson of the physical on our Earth. We will approach this process in a practical manner, using the knowledge of the masses, without judgment, but awash in love. With each example and every word the aura of love will provide an envelope around you and the words. This will help with the understanding and awareness which will broaden your perception as you read. This ability is common to the higher Spirit world. It is always used when high level Spirit Souls become involved in communication with Souls on Earth. This allows us to speak to the Soul memory rather than the ego self.

Evolved humans will learn the balance of body, mind and Spirit by starting first with the body. The tendency is great when we start on the path of evolution to concentrate on the Spiritual or the intellectual to the detriment of the physical. This needs to be reversed because the lessons of this age are many, and the physical strength and longevity are needed to be able to teach the masses. In the past, many very evolved Souls have had to leave their physical bodies before their missions were totally complete. They failed to maintain an awareness of the necessity of protecting the physical body.

In this moment in time, we are seeking once again the longevity of the physical body. This longevity will allow the intellectual mind and the Spirit of love and light to flourish to its full potential. Many Souls are dedicated to seeing our vision created and being a reality of Earth life. *The secret of joy at any time of the day is good health.* If we are in good physical health we stand a better chance of being in good emotional health. That does not mean that you will always react with emotional sadness to the experiences that happen in your life, but it does mean that you will be able to keep any and all disappointments in their proper perspective. You will be able to maintain that inward joy despite the circumstances that you experience physically.

Good health requires that we take care of our body and mind. Taking care of our body dictates that we eat the proper food, get enough sleep, exercise every day, and have a balance of work, play, and love in our lives. In addition to what we must give our body for health, there are additional rules of balance that require withholding chemicals of destruction. If we ignore one of these requirements, our daily world will not be in balance. Not being in balance can affect our physical, mental, and emotional health. We are an integrated unit of body, mind and Spirit. We cannot cheat any one part of ourselves and know the joy of health.

As a human being, our primary balance comes from the Earth. That is the way we chose it to be when we chose to be human. Being human focuses our primary point of reference within our Earth form. Therefore we cannot live without taking care of Earth's needs first. Our physical needs are proper food, air, water, sleep and exercise. Once we tend the garden of our body, we can focus on the garden of our thinking mind. Our mind requires work to be balanced. Work is defined as using the body and the mind. Work can manifest itself in an infinite number of forms. It is impossible for us to involve one part of ourselves without evolving the other parts. Any use of the body and mind that is directed for the good of human society can provide a balance. If it is not directed toward the overall good of the race, it will not keep our thinking mind balanced. The mind will always be somewhat off balance, regardless of the intellectual productivity, if the body is not balanced. In turn, the mind will also always be somewhat off balance, regardless of the intellectual productivity, if the Spirit is not balanced.

Contributions to human society take many forms and essentially cover most of our human efforts. This can be understood by the primary focus of our intention. If the primary focus is financial, rather than to serve humankind, then the intention is focused in a non-gratifying way for human satisfaction. The Earthly form of Spirit is manifested in love. Love can also take an infinite number of paths. Love, too, must always be directed for the good of humanity to provide a balance. Love is essential to our health. Love must be given and received. Love is a cycle. Love cannot go halfway. Love is the circle of energy that surrounds us to keep the unity of body, mind and Spirit well and functioning. Each integral part of the human form — body, mind and Spirit — influences the other parts. No one part can function without the other. There is an inherent integration of these essential parts of us. The influences of the body can clearly be seen as they impact on the mind and Spirit, the mind as it impacts on the body and Spirit, and the Spirit as it impacts on the body and mind. A failure to use any one part of self creates an imbalance of self.

As humans we need to look at each part of ourselves and see if we are balanced. In that internal observation we must be objective and willing to correct the imbalances that we may find. Correcting imbalances requires that we overcome the fear of change. The energy that we receive from the Universe is directed at each human being. If we are not balanced in any one part of ourselves we will have an energy block in that area. *The long-term effect of an energy block in our body is an illness or disease. This disease can manifest itself as a physical problem or emotional problem. In either case it is a disease of the body which is our physical point of reference on the Earth.*

In today's world there are those who focus strictly on one part of their BEING. They feel that their way is the true way of being human. It isn't. It is only their illusion. Illusions happen in life because of the challenges we are here to meet. No one can change another person's illusion. It is each person's private need. We can only change ourselves. If we fail to learn our lesson in this lifetime, there will be other times for us to return and work on the challenge again. There is no wrong or right way for us to choose to learn. There is only the experience that provides the lessons. *This book is for those who wish to open to the awareness and understanding that will allow them to see themselves and their roles in a different perspective.*

Many people at this moment in their evolution want to face their challenges with a broader perspective. Physical illness, as it is seen today, comes from both neglect and abuse of the body. We have lost our understanding of need for the physical body as the vehicle of our Spirit and Soul. The present Earth society has chosen the focus of intellectualism. Intellectualism is the opposing force to Spiritualism. Once a cycle is established it is very hard to change. Changing our belief system is a total relearning for us. Viewing the physical self and the diseases of self from the perspective of intellectual understanding gives us a distorted perception of the reality that we have created. We do not accept that we have any responsibility in the action of the total process of disease development.

Science has always searched for something or someone to blame, when we have disease of the mind or the body. Blaming becomes part of the disease, in many instances. We create our reality. We create the reality of disease with the action of our mind and the reaction of our body. We are what our illusion tells us that we should be. To understand disease, we must look at the illusion we create and the results of that creation. The first step to health is accepting responsibility for the creation of self. Every small physical imbalance is accepted today as a signal of death. Death is cloaked in fear because of other illusions. When we fear death, feel guilty and overcome with sin, accept that we can only look forward to hell and damnation when we pass on, it is natural from a human perspective to see a tiny pain as impending death.

Remember the illusion. We are told that "to sin is to suffer hellfire and damnation." We are told that "we are born with original sin." This is another illusion. The Spirit is not sadistic. We are living our hellfire and damnation through our own system of beliefs. We are creating our own "sin," based on the belief system that we have accepted within our world. Illusions are better known in our world as beliefs. Beliefs, of all varieties, begin to mold us the moment that we cry that first cry. Most are barbaric illusions that will never be. Unfortunately, we perpetuate illusions through the centuries in the form of religious teachings, intellectual concepts, cultural beliefs, dogma and "value" systems.

To look at each of these sources would require volumes. In this book I am focusing on the many influences of health only briefly, in an attempt to expand your awareness. We create our own world based on those beliefs that we have come to accept as truth, that control our thinking. We know no other way at the moment. The present energy movement on Earth is part of the Universal plan for the evolution of the human Soul. In order that we may evolve, we must be able to accept that our beliefs are illusions. An illusion is a false belief. Beliefs can be changed simply by understanding and exercising the free will of self to initiate change.

In time, our world will understand that life is change and that beliefs create the illusion of right or wrong. The belief in the concept of right and wrong places us in the position of judgment. One belief system that needs to be addressed first is the belief that we grow old, unhealthy, diseased and senile in the prime years of our life and proceed to a physical death. The marvelous mechanism of the body is so complex that it is not yet within a millennium of being understood. Today, the body is allowed to return to physical dust before it has hardly begun to live because we believe that we must die in a certain time frame. We are trapped in the world of illusion again. The truth is the body is capable of infinite life if it is balanced and productive, if it still has a goal to accomplish. Our belief is in retirement and old age as an inevitable part of maturity. This concept is not appropriate or productive to Soul evolution. Age is of the mind. The mind belief will force the body to respond to the belief as long as it exists. This is an example of the immediate and dramatic effect of the bridge that exists between the body and mind. At the time of physical death, there is rebirth of the eternal Spirit within the Spirit realm. Soon our Soul will consciously choose another Earth life. Without an awareness and understanding of the reality and purpose of Soul life, we will start from scratch again in each physical lifetime, learning the same things – within the same belief systems, with the same end result.

Is it any wonder that we need so many lives on Earth? Is it any wonder that it is time for an evolution in our awareness and understanding? For Soul evolution to be complete, we will need the guidance of many evolved Spirits who can challenge our perspective. This will lead to a change in the belief system and the teaching of love. Many Souls now on Earth have evolved to the level of seeking love. Do not be afraid to listen and feel. I will use the words, us, we, I, because you see I am part of you and you are part of me, we are all one in the Universe as energy. The actions of one become the actions of all, which allows us to understand the importance of growth and change in the energy we are living.

Looking at the belief system that contributes to the death of the physical body, we see many influences that are primary. The body should be a celebration of the mind and the Spirit. The body should be a communion of love and caring as the physical temple that it is. When we care about our body in the Spiritual sense and the intuitive sense, we will be offering it protection in the physical sense. In today's world, there is much that our body needs to be protected from.

Happiness is taking control of our life. That doesn't sound hard does it? Yet in our world happiness is perceived as difficult. The Universal Truth is all we have as our potential for living longer lives and happier lives.

With our present level of awareness and understanding we allow our belief system to control our entire physical world. Our ego is in charge of our physical body and our emotional health. The Joy of Health comes when we, as an integrated BEING, take charge of our physical body and our emotional health. There is no other way, if we want to experience health in the true sense of attunement with Nature. *Health is consciously controlling how we feel, how we think, and what we do. Health is always denying our belief system the right to control us as our thinking and behaviors.*

We are not the picture that our beliefs paint us to be; we are our unconscious, our inner self. We are love as the pattern of our emotional self, and we are designed as a vibrant physical being. When we care for our physical being as we were meant to care for it, as a part of Nature, we can consciously live in vibrant health until we have completed our work for this life on Earth and we consciously decide to leave. We can live in good health and productivity without disease for hundreds of years, once we can release our fear and our beliefs. This will decrease the number of times that we must return to this physical plane and start over, without Soul memory, to learn our eternal lessons as a human being.

Diseases are lessons of mental, emotional, and physical balance. Once this lesson is learned we have the freedom of health and a physical life which we control. When we have good physical health, our energy will be present for longevity. When we have good emotional health, our motivation will be present at multiple levels, and we will love our physical life. We need only to develop this awareness and understanding to guide us through each physical experience in the most productive manner. Our present age will have nothing to do with being able to progress, as I will outline in this book. Our body is in a constant state of regeneration. With our help it can be what we want it to be. Start right now with a thought in your mind of how you would like your physical self to be.

You are perfect just the way you are, but that is hard for your conscious mind to grasp and accept. We will strive, as we progress, to get your unconscious mind and your conscious mind into synchronicity, which allows them to work together as they trade off different aspects of learning. This will help with cellular regeneration. Your perfection comes from the Soul source as energy, not the physical source. The physical source is our present physical reality. Our point of power to change self is in the present moment. Therefore it follows, using both the rational mind and the unconscious mind, that we must protect our physical self if our power is to be at its maximum. We can do this. It does not work to ignore the physical body. Ignoring our temple requires that we spend endless hours on repair work and searching for solutions. The solutions are always within us and our memory – and so is the repairman if thoughts need to be cleaned up.

All disease is a result of either excesses or deficiencies. The excesses and deficiencies of life begin with the action of the mind and result in the reaction of the body. Many times this is experienced as too much improper food and too little proper food being provided for our body. The standard answer in the minds of many as they read this statement is, "I eat good food." My answer is, "Yes, you do eat food that tastes good, but is it good for your body?" Many people today understand this concept, but we are speaking to those who don't understand. Our taste buds are conditioned to like the food that we normally eat. Many people are not especially interested in change. That is the response of their externalized mind. Change will mean having your unconscious mind in synchronization with your conscious mind. Let me give you an example before we go further. In our society our car is a cherished possession. We have a hard time living without one. Because of this we will spend a large portion of our yearly income buying a car, maintaining the repair work, and feeding the car the precise fuel that will assure us of peak performance. When we feed our car we know that we will get the best performance with high-test gas and high-grade oil. We keep it lubricated regularly, and we wash it and we love it. We cannot conceive of mistreating our car, but we will routinely mistreat our physical body, which mistreats our thinking mind and loving emotions in the same way that it mistreats our sensory self. We may also mistreat other people without recognizing the absolute harm that we are inflicting upon them, simply because we have lost our chemical balance, and as we interact with other people, the interaction may not be perfect.

Yet every day we, as human beings, fail to provide the perfect food for our body. Many of us have a better relationship with our car than we have with our body. This may mean that our car will outlast our body's need for it. Death, as we believe in it, occurs in the middle years. This happens for many of us because we have abused our body. We do not see a way to fix it in our conscious mind so we simply make the decision to leave and develop a new life design. We make a Soul choice to abort our life design. We decide to physically experience death. Once we make this decision, we will unconsciously allow our human body to deteriorate, and sometimes we will be totally unaware of what we are doing to ourselves.

Unless we become aware of the physical lesson of Earth, we can spend many lifetimes dealing with the same old issue of learning to take care of our physical body. When we choose to be as considerate and appreciative of our body as we are of our car, we can enjoy life on Earth for an extended time. The focus of the physical self has been functioning from what I will term a commercial mentality for too many years. This mentality has created more diseases for us than has ever been known in the history of humankind. It creates materialism, fear, anger, guilt, greed, want, selfishness, over-developed egos, waste, starvation, gluttony, disease and physical death, yet for the most part we remain unaware of what is happening to us. This commercial mentality has de-vitaminized, de-mineralized and polluted our food supply until it is no miracle that pollution has in turn created a mammoth drug business. The drug pollution further poisons the physical self until there is sometimes no recognizable path leading back to a healthy body. This commercialism has become a way of life in our world. The belief in this system is so complete that we live in total fear of living without prepared foods. We know no other way that we can conceive of as being acceptable. We deny the responsibility for our own physical and emotional health when we accept this belief.

This fear creates a fear of immediate death if there is any indication of what appears to be a physical threat to the physical body. Pain in the body is equal to a problem in our car's engine. There is a problem with our fuel system and we have a significant buildup of waste material or the immediate fuel is inadequate. In either case we search for a mechanic, or a technician to repair the damage that we have created. Treating our pain with drugs or surgery are only temporary comfort measures. Many times they are measures that complicate the problem rather than solve it. The logical solution is to change our perspective of our body and the relationship it plays in our living.

What is high-test fuel for the body? The body's fuel should consist of 80% alkaline-forming foods and a maximum of 20% acid-forming foods. This will give us the organic mineral salts that are our biggest deficiency and our most needed food elements. Using this balanced fuel intake will restore our electromagnetic energy force. There is a generalized misunderstanding about foods in our society. The foods that we know as highly acid foods are alkaline-producing foods for the body. Foods that we see as alkaline foods are in reality acid-producing foods for the body.

The three groups of foods that are highly acid-producing within the body are fats, sugars and starches. These foods also provide the least in true nutrients to the body. Alkaline-producing foods are primarily fruits and vegetables with the exception of the highly starchy legumes which we need to monitor in quantity. Milk, fish, fowl and lamb are also partially alkaline-producing foods. The basic diet in our society consists of primarily the acid-forming foods. The deficiency of the organic mineral salts and other nutrients found in these acid-forming foods presents us with many of our current diseases, especially cancer and nervous system disorders.

The acid-forming foods allow the organisms found normally in our body to become virulent and produce countless infections. Most organisms will not flourish in an alkaline body. Our world is one of balance so it is important to eat of the partially alkaline-producing foods in addition to the fruits and vegetables. This provides our balance naturally and we do not have to concern ourselves with details. Fats are always acid-producing, and with the exception of those found naturally in the foods listed above, they should be avoided. In our society the fats, sugars and starches are some of our excesses.

More information on the foods that we should eat for health will be given later in this book. We need to attend to the foods that we eat, the air that we breathe and the water that we drink for the health of the body. These elements are the trilogy for physical health. As the body grows from infancy through the stages of physical development, the physical needs must be met. They will not basically change, but the contrast in what we supply in our world is worth noting. Understanding the need to properly care for the body will help us understand the development of body, mind and Spirit more fully as we live the periods of life.

The periods of life are clearly defined by what is known to the Universe as The Law of Sevens. I will discuss each period in turn as we cover the development of the physical self. All of life is divided into periods of seven years. This applies to the cellular structure as well as the developmental structure of the human form. Major changes will be evident to us in the year before and the year after these seven-year periods. Our external world will experience change and our internal world will experience change.

Look back at your life. Do you feel the same at forty that you felt at twenty? Do you believe the same things now that you believed thirty years ago? Has your understanding of life changed? Can you recognize these changes on a body, mind and Spirit level? Or, are you stuck in an old belief system that you should have outgrown? *Each period of life has its own individual purpose and collective purpose for being.* Each period experiences the influence of the bridges of integration that mold us into the total being of self to create the truth in our bridges of consciousness.

There is similarity in all and individuality in all. No two Souls will ever be totally the same, nor will they develop on exactly the same schedule. But for the purpose of clarity, the periods of life will be dealt with in the time frame of our physical reality. If you find yourself earlier than some periods and later in others, do not be alarmed, simply adjust to the information as your precise pattern. Some forty-year olds may find the pattern of their life to be younger or older than their physical age. This requires careful consideration because we should stay at our age level to keep ourselves from missing any part of our internal growth.

In the world of Spirit there is no time but our physical growth is divided into levels that we all must live.

THE HUMAN LESSONS OF THE UNIVERSAL LAW OF CREATION

SEVEN LEVELS

Law of Sevens

Law of Action and Reaction

Law of Cause and Effect

Law of Physical Balance

Law of Balance and Compensation

Law of Ethical Values- human energy lesson

Laws of Nature

We are one with Nature.

LAW OF SEVENS: **First Period**

In The Beginning, Our Physical Experience

In the beginning, the growth of the Soul in physical form is patterned by the Universal Law of Sevens. Growth of the physical body is also growth of the mind, emotions, and Sensory Spirit. They must be recognized as one unit in the human form. The Law of Sevens allows for a division of the growth periods with a special emphasis on the needs of the period. The Law of Sevens divides our life into seven-year periods that are calculated by our Spirit to be the precise time that we need to learn and to change from one level to the next level. These are called periods.

The first period of the Law of Sevens is the period of infancy. Infancy is the root establishment of the growth process of the three integrated units. This period is from birth to seven years, the first seven years of physical life. We will start with the food we give the body to allow for physical growth. Feeding of the body starts immediately from birth when the mother nurses the infant. This is Spirit's way to provide the perfectly balanced food which Spirit designed the mother's body to produce. It is the nectar of the Spirits. In this breast milk is all that an infant will need for the first few months of life. In addition to the nutrients, we have the mother's love and caring. The holding is the feeding of the Soul. The milk is feeding of the body.

Forego man-made milk in an infant's life. If the mother is not in balance and no milk comes, which is a true problem of imbalance in the health of the mother and her body, then feed the infant mother's milk from the mare or goat. This milk is the closest to the mother's nectar and will be easy for the infant to digest. It will allow the physical body to grow with few if any problems. Today's formulas do not work as well because of their chemical composition. The chemicals, fats, and sugars added to infant formulas establish a pattern within the cellular structure that can be the source of blockage in the energy flow. Babies are primarily energy that must also feed from the energy of the mother as they nurse.

After the first few months of an infant's life have passed the child can, if necessary, be placed on cow's milk. Cow's milk will be inferior unless food is added to the diet. Soybean milk, pure and without additions, is far superior to cow's milk for most infants. Cow's milk is hard for the human body to digest but is superior to those milks we make in our laboratories. Food should be added at the five-to-six month stage, depending on the infant's growth. If the child is large and hungry, he will need food in addition to milk at an earlier age. The mother will be told intuitively when this time is appropriate if she will listen.

An easy guide for the anxious parent: Know the foods of Nature and use them!

Added food should then be the food of Nature shared from the food of the family. It can be mashed to proper consistency without destroying its value. All food should be cooked without destroying its natural ingredients. This can be accomplished by steaming in racks or in patapar paper. Look to variety because deficiencies in diet cause deficiencies in health and the infant's growth. Know the foods of Nature and use them. They are an easy guide for an anxious parent.

While the mother is feeding her baby, her diet is crucial. Avoid the unnatural chemicals both during carrying and feeding because they can bring serious harm to the balance of the infant, just as they can bring serious harm to the balance of the mother. Eat from Nature in large quantities because you are eating for two, or three or more as the case may be. Nature's food will provide regularity to the mother's body, much milk for the little one, and a physical and emotional balance for the mother.

Truth is as truth does in feelings and in actions. Truth is the living Spirit of the human being. Healthy children are the result of healthy thoughts, healthy behaviors, and the physical practices of the mother and father of infants. They will be rewarded in healthy children with strong immune systems and strong mental and physical bodies. The infant senses the mother's emotions and mirrors them in his or her personality. Mothers that are at peace with themselves and their roles will have babies that are at peace with their new beginning. The handicaps will be few in a serene mother, unless there is an understanding on another plane for a sharing of a lesson. If that is the circumstance, the understanding will be there on an unconscious level and the inner peace will be there too.

Do not be nervous at the new role in your life. You chose to be a mother and you are worthy of the choice. Motherhood is another level in your evolution. We cannot evolve without the lessons for learning. All lessons come in the form of Earth experiences. Earth is our classroom. Do not be afraid to learn and to change with the flow of the energy vibrations of life. In the arrangements that have been made between infant and parent, you are the caretaker and the first and primary teacher for that Soul during this incarnation. The beliefs that you instill in this small being will influence it from birth and until death, but through maturity, it might gain another broader perception of the world around it, and of itself.

Those perceptions are many times won with extreme suffering, if the beliefs you teach are based in fear rather than love. The value system of the adult will be the value system of the infant, until another understanding is consciously learned. Therefore, the responsibility of the parent is more important than generally understood because the body, mind and Spirit is looking to that first teacher for guidance. All parts must have special attention if we are to be balanced. When this concept is better understood by parents, we will stop the wars, the killings and the fear which is so much a part of our society. We will also stop a large portion of the destructive behavior and habits that are learned in childhood.

In the beginning there was light. We present the darkness to ourselves. This is our illusion and is not a necessity of life. If there was a light in the beginning, we have obviously caused the darkness. As we evolve and begin to climb the stairs of Soul evolution, the lightness returns. In the lightness is JOY. Each moment that we raise our level of awareness in any of the integral parts of self we can feel JOY. Look inwardly now and find those moments within you. As a parent your first responsibility is to allow that infant to develop in the light of love. Love is the light. Fear is the darkness.

Do not cast a child into darkness. If that tiny Soul has spent other incarnations in darkness, you will be aware of your role of helping him/her to reach the light on an unconscious level. Do not let this responsibility frighten you. Spirit does not allow you to accept a challenge if you have no chance of success. Different lifetimes will be devoted to different challenges for each of us. Each life is full of multiple lessons. Part of our lesson is to accept the responsibility for the challenges that we have chosen and stay detached from those that are not ours. It is part of our human personality to covet what isn't ours and resist what is.

When we reach the point of perfect balance with body, mind and Spirit, the resistance fades away. At that moment we will find ourselves in the flow of our own reality – accepting and loving. Loving the infant is a bonding of that concept in the child's Earth consciousness. On the Earth level this is identified as a love bond between parent and child. A love bond does truly exist, but it is our actions that are computed by an infant's senses. The physical senses compute the action of love or fear and that perception becomes the basis of that child's reality. The infant is sensitive to the vibrations of energy that the parents or other individuals release around him. This energy does not have to be directed towards the infant, but the energy of the space will be absorbed and understood by the Soul of the infant. In infancy the five physical senses develop soon after birth. The physical senses are acute definers for the tiny one after leaving the womb. Do not believe that the infant is too young to understand the vibrations of energy.

We begin to teach by the energy vibrations that we create. The energy created becomes the action created. Energy is the living Spirit of action. All energy and all actions need to be based in love. We start from the beginning to teach love to this infant Soul that has joined us here on Earth. In this respect, organized religion has fallen short of Spirit's plan. Centuries back, in the evolution of Earth, we decided to focus on fear, guilt and sin in the teaching of the churches. We conceived and enforced this way of maintaining control of the followers. That has not been and is not now a part of Spirit's plan. The concept of Spirit has always been love. In the beginning there was light. At the moment of birth we are light. We create the darkness.

The time has come for the church teachings to revert from the focus of fear to the focus of love. As humans we have begun to have a better understanding of love as the truth of self and life. In teaching love Spirit meant infinite love, love of all, including love of Spirit and

Self because Spirit is in each of us as our energy pattern of love. If we fail to love each other and ourselves, we fail to love Spirit. We are each living in our Spirit Energy as the reflective presence of the overall Spirit Energy. The infant is the Spirit's living presence in total innocence, and as older and wiser parents, we are the teacher of love to our infant children. If we fail to teach love, we teach by acting out the opposite of love, which is fear. Said in another way, if we fail to teach light, we teach darkness. If parenting is allowed to flow naturally, allowing the infant its natural flow of growth and change with the support of your love, the child will maintain the light of love. Love is the only requirement for light.

The Three Primary Energy Forces of Our Thinking Mind

A Soul that focuses on love, loves all people including self. It knows no other way. Darkness has not entered its consciousness, therefore it cannot know fear. Allowing an infant to thrive in the abundance of love will quickly develop the awareness of intuition, intellect, and rational thought in the child. These are the three primary energy forces of the thinking mind. The Spirit is life, the Soul mind is the builder, and the body is the result. It is with the beliefs of our thinking mind that we build the body. If we fail to begin this life with love then we can create chaos in the development of our physical body. Our body always serves as a reflection of our thinking mind. The transmitted feelings, emotions, and actions of adults influence the building blocks of the mind of the infant.

The beliefs and the physical behaviors that we live always influence the thinking minds of our children and thus we create carbon copies of our challenges in our children. If the parent is in darkness, darkness is created within the Soul of the infant. Scientists have spent fortunes researching the hereditary influences of disease on Earth. Disease is not as dependent on the genetic pattern as it is dependent upon the belief system, especially our beliefs about food and our lifestyle. If an infant grows up with parents who are suffering from a disease (choose your own disease), that infant is mentally patterned to have the disease unless his awareness develops to the point of understanding his own creation and how to avoid that specific illness. Developing the disease will create the illusion of a hereditary disease because the belief will be passed through the family in the same manner as the antigens.

The medical profession has supported, indeed has created, the concept of hereditary disease. This is an established scientific belief in the concept of disease creation. This concept has placed the stamp of scientific credibility on the individual to create the disease. Medical statistics become self-fulfilling prophecies more surely than the predictions of a seer. We could say that what we see and how we live is the way that we create ourselves.

The mother's milk starts the infant in the process of physical growth. As the infant reaches the fifth or sixth month of life it is important to begin adding Nature's foods. As was true with the mother's milk, which is Nature's food for the infant, we need to continue with Nature's food for the child. Infancy blends into childhood as the child grows and develops. A child is a maturing infant, so time again is an issue and will be left to the mother's intuition. As the food is added it needs to consistently be the food of Nature. Do not let this be commercial food with chemicals, for the influence on the infant will be to lower the system of resistance within the body, plus a failure to replace the necessary chemicals that create good health, which allows disease to be prevalent in the child's life.

While the mother is nursing, she should eat from Nature's food. When the infant eats, he should eat from Nature's food. The pure foods of Nature will provide fewer man-made chemicals than processed food. They will also provide the needed mineral salts and nutrients that will protect the infant and allow its physical development. Our society begins the introduction of processed food at the moment that food is presented. If the infant is not fed from the mother's milk, polluted food begins at birth. If the infant is fed from the mother's milk, then polluted foods are started at the moment that the introduction of other foods begins. It does not take long in today's society to have the child eating from our so-called "fast food," which weakens the child's immune system. When food is introduced, it should be as chemically free as we can provide. This can happen if the infant is fed food from a family table of healthy food. Of course, if the entire family is being fed polluted food, it is time to reevaluate the quality of food for everyone. It is time to examine the belief system and to see how carefully the entire family is eating from Nature.

This period of development depends upon the constant replenishing of the organic mineral salts that come from Nature. This is a crucial period in physical and mental development. The human body is designed to assimilate the mineral salts that occur organically in the Earth. When the mother eats of the foods from Nature, she provides these important minerals to the infant through her milk. Human milk can provide what an infant needs for many months, but there will come a time when the stress will be too great for the mother, and the child can be switched to table foods. Infants who are fed from commercial preparations will find it more difficult to avoid our society's illnesses. They will need the introduction of table foods much earlier. They will thrive better when these foods are grown organically and cooked properly. Foods should be cooked with as little decrease in their nutrients and mineral salts as the mother can manage. Once an infant has been placed on normal food, the quality of that food will determine his health and his physical resistance to disease. When love is added to the goodness of food, the energy of the body will be at its peak in protective response. There is no other way. The food that you give the infant is the food that is responsible for the growth of the total cellular structure of the physical body, and the entire nervous system including the brain, which will be with the child for its entire lifetime.

If you feed the infant fats, starches, and sugars primarily and very few fruits, vegetables and quality protein, then he will live with an acid base to his cellular system, which will interfere in the physical growth process. This acid base will make him more susceptible to the growth of the "germs," which he will breathe in the air around him. You will have a sick infant and a sick child. When the mother is still breast-feeding, the correct balance will be easier to maintain. Once breast milk is no longer supplied to the infant, the food that is fed to him is responsible for his entire cellular growth and chemical balance. Infants and children who eat large amounts of sugars and fast foods will begin their health problems early. Some will show symptoms of this early in life, others may not, but the damage will be in progress internally. It may take fifteen, twenty-five or forty years, but it will eventually create a physical problem.

Eating the wrong foods early in life establishes the unhealthy habit patterns and perpetuates the concept that all food is good food. An infant that learns to eat improperly may never know, as an adult, the significance of the proper foods or have any concept or awareness that there is a difference. The concept of food is a cultural concept. Being a cultural food does not mean that it is the proper food for the growth of the body, or that the food is organically grown. Some of the older cultures had better eating habits and fewer fatal diseases before they were influenced by the current fast-food culture. In our current American culture the average person, even the young child, is primarily living a dependency upon processed and/or fast food. This pattern of eating does not improve the body or mind of the infant who grows up eating "fast food" exclusively or often. The body learns to change some essential nutrients into the chemicals that are essential but are not provided in some foods. Therefore if some of the right foods are consumed the body will adjust, to a degree, for a short period of time. Those infants at high risk are those who are deprived of all food that might provide some of the essential nutrients that are necessary to human growth.

Alcoholism and drug addiction are the results of tremendous imbalances within the body, many times starting from infancy and childhood, only to be acted out in the teens and twenties. Physical imbalances produce mental imbalances, as well as establishing addictive needs within the cellular system. Creating chemical imbalances during the most important school years can be an intellectual and emotional disaster. Infants and children with high sugar intakes will be imbalanced and the body will react in several different ways. Hyperactivity of childhood is a problem of sugar and chemical intake. This will be dealt with later by the body craving alcohol and drugs that can mimic a simple carbohydrate or sugar craving. When this pattern has been established, the body will respond to its feeling of need. Not only has the infant's body been conditioned, but the infant's mind has been conditioned. Addiction is the next step, and the combination will interfere in the physical future of the child.

Addiction will be dealt with later in this commentary, but at this point it is important to understand that a habit of non-disciplined intake has been established with addiction. The physical response to this high sugar intake can take many forms. In some infants, it will be diabetes. In others it will be alcoholism, drug addiction, obesity, or numerous other emotional and physical diseases that will happen in their later life. *Nothing can ever be more important to the infant and child than the food they eat and the love they receive.* These are foods of equal value. Many who pay hours of attention to the loving do not understand that love is also in the actions, especially in the eating, drinking, and breathing of that young child. The action of preparing the proper foods for the body and withholding improper foods is an act of love, not punishment. We are consciously denying a habit that will last a lifetime and have a tremendous influence upon that life if we do not teach our children by our own personal actions. Food processors are in business to make money, not to cure disease, and not to prevent disease. For many years our American culture has been hypnotized into believing that processed food and fast foods are the answer to everything from our breakfast to our bedtime snack. Frequently this behavior leads to a lifetime of malnutrition, which can create diseases early in life. We are what we eat!

All food is good food is an illusion that has led many of us into our own illusion of saving time and money by eating inferior foods. What we are doing is preparing our body for an early old age and possibly death from disease. As parents we have the choice of nutrition to present to our growing infant. That teaching will be significant because it will affect our children from infancy to death if their level of awareness about eating does not change as they become aware of the options of free choice. The body's cellular structure is constantly changing, and within a seven-year period the cells have regenerated if we eat properly. Anyone who has the motivation of Spirit and the understanding of healing within the mind can restore his/her physical body to health and vitality if it is afflicted with disease.

A parent can do much to restore health to an infant by the devoted care of proper feeding. It will always work if done with persistence and love. From infancy through childhood a parent is presented with a blank slate in the functional mind of their progeny. It is the perfect time to teach the young child in the ways of health and healing. An infant can easily be taught the art of healing and eating properly. Many infants will return to a new life with a distinct memory of good foods and the joy of eating. During the period of infancy Soul memories are predominant and can be encouraged. These Soul memories can encompass many thousands of lifetimes. The information is there to be used. This is more challenging as a teaching for today's parents because they were not taught this concept of past life memory from our physical past lives. Those parents who learn and teach a child to explore their Soul memories will parent a new generation of adults on Earth. Understanding our mode of creation will help us create on a different level for ourselves, our children and our friends. We are all teachers. In our actions we display the patterns of our mind and Soul. Honor the infants in your midst. They are holy creations and they are our pupils.

Involved in the concept of responsibility for infants and children is the responsibility of self. Health is of the body, mind, and Spirit. It is the balance of each energy field that allows the energy to flow through the contact points of our physical being and ground us to the Earth. We are part of Nature. We are an element of Nature, the same as the trees, flowers, fruits, vegetables, animals and all living creatures. We have all been placed on this Earth for a definite purpose. We are here to flow into the rest of Nature's abundance, and it is through

Nature's abundance that we find our physical, mental, and emotional strength.

This is why we do better spiritually, mentally and physically when we eat only from Nature's abundance. To eat from the abundance of the place where we are living provides additional vibratory waves of energy for greater balance and grounding. Greater balance speeds Soul evolution, preserves the body, and expands the mind in all three forces. The ingestion of foreign chemicals into the body interferes with the vibratory response of the cells. This faulty vibration will affect every cell within the body. It puts into motion a discord that vibrates throughout the entire physical, emotional and Spiritual systems. This discord, when joined with the belief system, converts the cellular energy into disruptive energy or negative energy blocks which, with time, develop into destructive (dark) energy or disease. This discord can be set in motion through chemicals, beliefs, processed foods, medications, fear, anger, guilt and hate (all dark or negative emotions), creating negative energy.

The Cellular Concept of Behavioral Conditioning

Our cells are patterned by us and respond to our chemical commands, which come from our behaviors, thinking, emotions, eating, drinking, and breathing. This is the cellular concept of behavioral conditioning, which in our scientific world is a mental approach. But in reality we are one, as energy and matter. Each integral part has a like concept. Our physical body dies and is recreated over and over again during each incarnation from the energy of our Spirit Consciousness. Cells die and are replaced on a daily basis. In a seven-year span we are physically new again for the early years of our life.

If we can understand this concept we can understand that senility is a product of our behaviors and belief system. This will allow us to understand that no one dies until they are ready to do so. The more advanced Souls will choose to live longer in the future as they shed their belief system, and learn to balance their physical bodies. We cannot live without the physical body on Earth. Our Spirit never knows death. Only our physical body experiences death. Increased awareness of the thinking mind allows us to build a body to suit our needs. *Building a body is a day to day creation of health rather than neglect or abuse. Health is a personal responsibility.* Consistent abuse is an unconscious need for disease and death. Abuse is an unconscious action of self-hate, and we routinely heap abuse upon ourselves with our thinking, emotions, and behaviors.

Building of the body begins at conception. This first period of Earth existence for us is laying the foundation for the remainder of our physical lives. We are placing our building blocks. We will use these building blocks in the continued growth of our body, mind and Spirit. There is no other way. We start creating our reality the moment we are born. The Soul that enters as an infant is aware of the lessons of its life. The understanding of these lessons starts to dissolve gradually as the belief system is being structured. The older the child becomes the more clouded its choice of lessons will become. We must learn to consciously keep the channels open to the infant Soul memories. Our world is becoming better at this.

An infant will be in constant communication with the Universal Consciousness. Communication is a reality through infancy but starts to fade during the years from four to seven. Parents should encourage the child to stay open to the Spirit Communication of his world. This communication needs to be understood and supported. Communication with the Souls of friends and loved ones does not mean that the child needs to see a psychiatrist. The child must be supported in understanding the normal Spirit communication that he is capable of living on Earth as a direct reflection from his past human lives. Open-mindedness is a trait to be cherished and consciously preserved. Starting from birth is the ideal time and place. Picking up these lessons in mid-life becomes a challenge within itself. Releasing a firmly planted belief system is the challenge to understanding life in the adult mind. Cherish our infants, love them, communicate with them and allow them the freedom of expression. This does not mean that the adults must be controlled by the child. A disciplined structure should be provided in which they can feel safe in being their own imaginative selves. Discipline and structure are truly physical manifestations of love. We should all love our children, and guide them into a loving adult life. This first period of growth for the body, mind and Spirit is the beginning of the physical sojourn.

LAW OF SEVENS: **Second Period**

Childhood, Learning the Fine Art of Being a Sensory Being

The second period of the Law of Sevens is the time of childhood. This period is from the beginning of the eighth year through the end of year fourteen. It is the continuation of the growth process of all three units of self. During this period there is an acceleration of understanding. Curiosity about the self and the Universe are forces that are developing in the period of childhood. These intellectual forces are combined with the development of understanding, making this an extremely valuable time for positive influences for the child.

Each period of life responds to its influences and molds the growth for that period. None is more important than the next. In each period, the Soul knows its responsibility for continued evolvement. When the subconscious finds itself in other than positive influences, it will encourage testing on the conscious level. There are several characteristics that must be patterned by the parents during the first three periods of life. This child is a new physical being. The child will be developing the physical senses, which will be the design for learning in this first period. They will learn by what they see, what they hear, what they touch, what they smell and what they taste. In addition to the physical senses, the infant and child are in command of their unconscious or Spiritual senses. They feel, see, and respond to the energy vibrations of actions, thoughts, sounds, tastes, smells and sights. They are learning the fine art of being a sensory being.

Children start at birth and continue through their entire life to learn by observation of action. Imitation is a strong force during the first three periods of life. Words will consistently teach less than action. As a parent we cannot say one thing, while we are being and doing another thing. At this age visual and sound teaching are more profound for the memory, although words are extremely important. It is the combined energy force of the five senses that is manifested in the attitude and personality of the child.

The characteristics that need to be observed and heard are those of love, truth, honesty, faithfulness, trust, patience, tolerance, gentleness, joy, defenselessness, non-judgment, generosity, wisdom, and open-mindedness. Mastering love as the first level will help with all the others (see the list of Ethical Values at end of book). A child who grows in the presence of unconditional love will automatically absorb the love plus all of the other caring traits, because they will be there, in their journey of life, to observe and copy as a means of learning. Beliefs, behaviors and motivation are patterned in childhood by what is seen and what is heard. This can frequently be seen manifested in body image and body language. You are the master of the body, mind and Soul as the parent. Silent messages and psychic messages are easily understood in childhood, but not usually on a conscious basis. Because of this, you must BE what you appear to BE or a child will know the difference. This understanding, even when it is not discussed, is profound and meaningful in a child's development process. *Always talk to your children.*

During this period significant changes can be seen in physical appearance. Cells change constantly, with seven years being the maximum life span for any cell. Cells restructure by ancient memory patterns. During the first three periods, the memory patterning is not as thoroughly formulated. Without a clear definition of memory, the cells reform according to the energy around them which they absorb. Children developing in positive energy may change from ugly ducklings to beautiful children, and the opposite can also happen. This is the physical effect of love. The physical effect can be observed in the same way that the behavioral effect can be observed. Children are what they are taught to be. The physical effect of love may be observed at any time in our life. Have you ever observed the beauty of a woman in love? Many people are conscious of the radiant "glow" emanating from a pregnant woman.

Love has the power to change the appearance of the physical self. The love that is bestowed upon a child affects the beauty of the child. Happiness and joy will shine in the physical body of anyone who is living in the energy of love. During this period teaching includes caring for self, as an example of the needs and self-love that each of us should give to ourselves. The physical body is in a period of extensive growth during this period of development. Cellular growth requires our replenishing the elements of Nature. These important natural elements can only come from the foods of Nature. Eating properly in this period is essential.

The child is the original Mime.

It is during the first and second periods of growth from infancy that eating habits are established. Our old saying, "Monkey see, monkey do" is appropriate. The child is the original mime. We cannot teach a child effectively, unless we can do as we teach. The second period is a period of learning habits that develop lifetime lessons. Addictive behavior is commonly learned during this second period. Addictive behavior does not have to refer to the ingestion of drugs or alcohol as most of our world views it. Addiction describes a "pattern of life" that can be good as well as bad, and it is imperative that we see good addictions as appropriate and "bad" addictions as inappropriate. We can all have addictions to good patterns as well as "bad" patterns.

Inappropriate addictive behavior is when we find ourself on a course that we refuse to change, despite the recognition that the behavior is destructive to us. This addictive behavior may be found in relationships, physical behavior such as violence, judgment, eating, drugs, alcohol, disease or any one of our many beliefs. Addiction is the opposite of open-mindedness. With addiction we are locked into a concept. We have the ability to change any belief and any behavior if that is our choice. But if it is not our choice, we are living without motivation. We fail to look at ourself and admit that the true problem is and has always been us. Know how you are thinking, and what change means to you. We frequently refuse to learn and to change. It is a human trait to want to suffer, not a Spiritual trait. It is common for us to become addicted to a belief system, another person, eating, drinking and drugs. Addiction is a singular focus, a closed mind. It is the opposite of open-mindedness, which we must use if we want to understand ourselves and our focus in life. Each Soul chooses the people that will influence his/her teachings before birth. A parent's capabilities are understood by the Soul when the Soul makes its choice to be their child. Each Soul has free will, the will of choice and intent, from birth. Having free choice means there are always alternatives available to the Dual Soul.

During childhood the choice of the parents can affect the choice of the child. All choices are integrated with lessons to be learned. Nothing is essentially wrong. It is simply a choice. The lesson for the child may be more difficult if the parent chooses a path other than the path agreed upon prior to birth. That does not make the choice wrong. The lesson is still there for both parent and child, but it is being approached from a different perspective. If the lesson is not learned in this lifetime, it will become Karma for the next lifetime. Karma is not punishment; it is the completion of an old Dual Soul lesson.

Bringing children into the world with love and teaching them love will make their physical lessons easier. Life is our classroom on Earth. As a student in school, we are promoted to the next level of study with different courses once we learn the lesson we are currently studying. Life is the same. Earth is the school of life. Life is the classroom. We visit many classrooms during the entire duration of academic education, which covers the entirety of all physical lives, and all Dual Soul lives. In life we visit many classrooms in our learning process, and when we resist learning we must live the lesson over and over again until we understand precisely what we are attempting to teach ourselves.

The Soul advantage in positive learning is not spending the time repeating the lesson. The Soul purpose for each of us on Earth is learning to BE in the perfection of Spirit. *In the Spirit World, Spirit is defined as the positive energy of life.* The lessons are Universal but our dramas for learning are individualized. Despite being individualized, the learning is the same. The travels of the Soul are mirrored in our travels as human beings.

We call this trip "life."

If I decided to make a trip from my home in Pittsboro, NC to San Diego, CA, there are many roads that I could take by car, there are many planes that I could take by air, there are buses, there are trains or I could choose to walk. I would be faced with choosing a method and a route. I would have many alternatives. I would make my choice based on the physical and mental concepts of the moment. When my Soul travels through the learning process, it has many choices. The Soul choice will be made according to the needs of the Soul. Every Soul begins a cross country trip at the moment of birth, which it lives until the moment of death. We call this trip "life." When you hear a story from a friend about some drama of life, you will always be able to find the threads of similarity for you in the lesson even if the dramas are totally different. Listening with awareness of this message will help you on a conscious level with your own lessons. This is one level of teaching and learning. If you were on your way to a shopping center and the announcer on the radio informed you that one of the roads you planned to take was now closed, you would make another choice. We are always receiving messages of help, with that "best" choice usually coming from our Spirit Consciousness.

Those who have made the choice not to possess the capability of seeing and hearing will need much longer to learn, but they are working on awareness from the level of sensing and feeling. These Souls are many times advanced Souls who are developing their total consciousness through both the past and the present. Many of them may choose not to communicate at all during this learning period. This is also a method used by Souls who wish to only experience emotion. All of life is a lesson; therefore, we have physical lessons with an emotional component, which helps us to learn the lesson from many different energy images of life.

Muteness can also be a choice for a child who finds the energy to be such that he feels unable to accomplish his lesson during this lifetime by talking. Death can also be a choice under such circumstances. This does not mean that the circumstances are wrong - it only means that they may not match the lesson chosen by this evolving Dual Soul. The lesson may be the muteness, or the death experience itself. Once we understand that all of life includes death and many other experiences, we can begin to see that nothing in life is right or wrong.

Some Souls will come to Earth for only brief periods, choosing to die in infancy or childhood. This is their choice, or their immediate lesson. It is important for us as parents to understand that even an infant controls its life span, if that is his wish. Children who are abused and die agreed to participate in the lesson with the other involved Soul. The lesson could be different for both Souls but it was their individual lesson. Those who die young came with specific lessons to learn. When those lessons are learned, they will leave this incarnation on Earth. They have completed their plan. The parent is aware of the plan and has agreed to participate on a subconscious level, which does not abort the grief of the Soul from the loss of the child.

Most Souls choose to learn a series of lessons with each incarnation. It may be the same series repeated over and over for many lifetimes for them. Or perhaps there are a few changes, but all lessons must be learned before they can be dropped from our human drama of life. Advancement of the Dual Soul can be somewhat, though not entirely, defined by the focus of the Dual Soul on Earth. There are levels that aware people can use to detect an advanced Dual Soul.

How to Detect an Advanced Soul

This is beneficial for making friends in our physical world. For instance, an advanced Soul who speaks only the truth will not enjoy being around someone who doesn't speak the truth. An advanced Soul will be uncomfortable around a person who curses, smokes, drinks and lavishes in sexual escapades. The energy will not be an energy that is comfortable for either party. The combined energies of advanced Souls free the energy and strengthen it for purposes of learning and creativity. It is a true advantage to be in the presence of, or to be loved by an advanced Soul. You will be in a positive energy stream that will make you feel good. Detection of the advanced Soul is possible by observation of their light energy and the way that they live their lives. There will be a peace and joy that can be felt, wherever they are.

For those Souls who are aware of light, look for joyful, positive and truthful behavior. Those Souls who live in negative energy are Souls who are still learning the basic lessons in Soul evolution and can be found living negative lessons. Souls who consciously or unconsciously focus on the positive such as love, caring, creating, sharing, honesty, responsibility and joy are the advanced Souls. Any Soul that is living in self-judgment is going to attract judgment from other people, which, if the Soul listens carefully, can be very helpful. Recognition is necessary for grouping of these Souls into advanced energy streams. These focuses will be present from childhood but the individual Soul awareness will vary. This energy is retained Soul experience and it is present in each and every Soul regardless of the level of awareness. Awareness itself will change with growth. Parents dealing with their children during the periods of infancy and childhood should always be aware of and encourage Soul memory. Soul memory leads to a greater understanding and awareness of the Earth lessons and a more rapid evolvement of the Soul. During infancy and childhood the senses are acute on all levels of consciousness.

The conscious level for the human is the mind level. The unconscious level for man is the Spiritual level. The subconscious level is the Soul memory level. The physical consciousness level is the physical sensory level.

This is the perfect time to teach discipline, structure, nutrition, healing, love, equality and all the positive characteristics necessary to Soul development. All new teachings will be integrated with all previous learning, making each individual a more aware human being.

It is also at this time that parents must remember a child operates from more than their five physical senses. They are operating from all levels of consciousness. They are picking up more energy vibrations than you are consciously picking up. Children learn and react to these vibrations which we and others send out. BE love, BE positive and you will have a loving, positive child. The belief system is not yet a force to be overcome during this period of development. The slate is clean and open. Taking advantage of the open-mindedness of children is a valuable gift, if done in a positive and loving manner, and it helps the adult understand more about themselves. Many children evolve with little or no structure or discipline provided by the parents.

A child learns love, security and respect for other Souls through discipline, structure and positive teachings. Discipline and structure are true guidance and teaching. They are not abusive behavior. Not providing discipline and structure is not providing love. It is a failure to care adequately about the development of the Soul who chose you as a parent. What we create in the life of another person, we will create in our own life as a means of learning. Learning discipline and structure helps with the

Soul focus throughout life. The Soul focus is impossible without discipline and structure. Without this loving guidance and teaching, the Soul will grow up by picking up fragments of knowledge in a helter skelter manner, which usually in our society means they will seek their knowledge "on the street." The thinking mind will not focus and learn to structure the living as a growth potential. This Soul will spend a life of fragmentation. The openness of childhood speeds the process of learning and gets the Soul off to a good start.

Structure and discipline teach the child how to operate successfully in the physical world. We would not expect a young adult to climb into the cockpit of a super jet and fly it to Europe without first learning how to be a pilot. If the child created this behavior from past life memory, the event could be successful. If we fail to teach a child structure and discipline, we are expecting them to fly in the world of life without learning how to cope with life. If we have not learned to cope with life from other lifetimes, then we must learn to cope with life so that it becomes second Nature within our memory.

In the fast-paced society of Earth, not enough nutrition is taught to children by example. Fast food, as we call it, has become a way of life, especially for the parents of small children. This example of inadequate food consumption is learned as the acceptable way, the fun or convenient way of eating. This lesson will lead to lessons of disease in life. The lessons of disease are time-consuming and often require a new entrance to Earth. This is why it behooves us to learn all of our lessons well, especially the lesson of nutrition. Caring for our physical body is an Earth lesson. It is only through the physical that we have power on Earth.

The first rule of being human is we must have a physical body. With a healthy physical body we can stay on Earth long enough to learn the lessons that we have come here to learn. There is no other way. Each human being is an evolved Spirit Energy living in a human physical body. Not every human is living from the same level of Spiritual Evolution. Disease is, in one respect, the Karma of poor nutrition. If the physical lesson is not learned we will keep repeating it with each incarnation. When we understand this lesson as human beings, there will no longer be a need for disease. Learning the lesson of caring for our body as a child can give us a better quality of time to learn other lessons. Many Souls have become attached to this Karma of disease, and they cannot see the lesson that they have designed for themselves to live. Therefore, many Souls on Earth spend a lifetime struggling with disease.

A child is open to the lesson of body, mind coordination and can be taught this lesson from the beginning of life. Many incarnations are spent on the Soul lesson of physical health. This is necessary because of the unity of body, mind and Spirit. We are three distinct parts and types of energy as a human being. One part cannot function at an optimum level without the other parts. As a human being we are indeed an integrated whole. The physical lesson must be learned in the first step of the consciousness as the total integration process.

In the first three periods of life, when physical growth is the major focus, the nutritional intake and teachings are vital to the rest of the present sojourn of life. Saying "eat right" to a child and then taking them to a fast-food restaurant is teaching the wrong message by action. Believe me when I tell you that the action was more quickly learned from behavior than your words. The "eat right" theory, even if defined, has become meaningless. Children grow into adulthood and believe that eating fast food IS eating right. It will take many years and countless hours spent worrying about disease before this teaching is reversed in the memory pattern of humanity.

"Eating Right"!

Eating right is the same for all periods of life. Eating right is eating from Nature! This covers the span of life from birth to death. Infants who eat from Nature start with mother's milk and soon progress to grains, fruits, vegetables and meats. This is the pattern that should be continued for life – in all periods. As habits develop, children are taught to eat excessive amounts of sugars, starches, and fats. These foods are detrimental to the body, especially when processed by human concepts and consumed in large quantities. Lean meats have value, natural sugar and natural starch have value, as they are consumed from Nature's provisions in the proper quantities. Fats, sugar and starch consumed as processed food become the excesses of eating. Anyone who chooses these foods as his/her primary daily diet is choosing the lessons of disease. There is no other way!

This choice of processed foods is eating from "the tree of knowledge" rather than eating from Nature's bounty. Spirit has provided man with natural food for the natural evolution of body, mind and Spirit. When we are presented with a choice in food, and make the conscious decision to consume de-vitaminized, de-mineralized, non-fibrous food that has been polluted with man-made chemicals, fats, sugars and starches that are superfluous to the food the body needs, we are consciously choosing the path of a lesson in disease.

The body will not promote or allow the growth of organisms in an alkaline-balanced body. Eating from Nature's bounty will automatically assure us of essentially 80% alkaline-producing foods and 20% acid-producing foods, if we eat a variety of Nature's foods. The percentages will vary from time to time and body to body, but the variance will usually be acceptable and healthy. The waste products of this diet will be cared for naturally by the body, without harmful effects. Nature is the path of health and well-being. This is the path that will allow the opening of the mind and Spirit. We cannot fully develop the mind and Spirit, without first understanding the role of the physical body. Understanding the role of the body allows for true vital living. It allows for viability of total cellular structure and function, which includes the energy development of the mind, body, and Spirit. The choice belongs to each of us as individuals.

The food that a child eats and the loving energy that surrounds him determine the number of illnesses that the child will experience. Some of Nature's foods are germicidal within the body. The most important of these foods is the orange, but all citrus fruits are beneficial. Different fruits and vegetables have this germicidal capability, because of their natural chemical composition. Eating these foods raw retains their natural properties. The electromagnetic energy contained within raw food cannot be obtained in any other way.

Any child can and should be taught to eat oranges and other fruits frequently in infancy and in childhood. Eating oranges and drinking fresh orange juice will assure any Soul of a healthier body. An infant should be fed fresh orange juice with a spoon, starting as early as one month. The many viral diseases that plague children in our world today are the result of an improper alkaline-acid ratio within the body. Natural fruit acids are highly alkaline within the body, and prevent the growth of opportunistic organisms that are the source of our diseases. Disease is a combination of the excesses and deficiencies that we subject our physical self to on a consistent basis. These excesses and deficiencies are not all food, alcohol and drugs. They also include any obsessive thoughts, actions or negative beliefs. Anyone who lives in fear, hate, and anger will have a body response that will be dis-ease or disease.

Infants and children who are fed primarily processed food and fast food will be susceptible to various problems from hyperactivity to fatal illnesses. These young bodies must deal with an improper balance, waste material and chemicals, before the body is mature enough. The child will have many disadvantages to survival under such conditions. Ear infections, strep throat, and bladder infections will be constant irritations, as will arthritic conditions. Their life will be a drama of excesses and deficiencies first in nutrition and then in pain of the body, mind and Spirit. The lesson of nutrition, if not learned by good example, becomes thoroughly misunderstood and improper eating habits are established as part of the belief system, through observed actions.

There are two lessons here. Parents are put in the position of dealing with childhood illnesses that seem to be endless as they learn the lesson of nutrition. This causes additional stress and worry to be added to what each Soul sees as his/her own individual problems. Sick children become a true lesson in patience and discipline for the parents, as well as a lesson in nutrition and disease for both the parent and the child. Always entwined in the lessons of disease are a multitude of related lessons. These are primarily physical lessons that are there to be learned first, before the mind and Spirit can be truly creative. But the lessons of patience, inner peace, tolerance, understanding, and love can be lessons that Souls work through in the process of having diseases and having children with disease.

Developing the Body through expansion of the Mind

The second period of life is a period of development of the body through the expansion of the mind. It is a period of establishing habits and formulating beliefs from what you see and what you hear. It is a period of learning the excitement of discipline and structure, whose groundwork was started in the first period. Without this early learning we cannot easily understand the focus of Soul evolution as a later focus of life. From birth to seven years the slate is fairly clean. From eight to fifteen it begins to fill rapidly. The teachings become beliefs. We act out from our beliefs for a lifetime. The circumstances of our physical reality find their basis of creation during these first two periods of life.

Self-Evaluation Exercise

It is valuable in Soul development to review our memory of these two periods. Every happening, every word has a Soul meaning, a Soul influence. Reviewing is not judgment, it is review. Looking at anything with judgment will prevent us from seeing. Evaluation of self and others must always be done with discernment, not judgment. The purpose is to understand the reality, the fact, not to make that fact right or wrong. Review for: reaction to, beliefs from, and perception of. Doing this review will expand our understanding of why we are, who we are. This can be our beginning of bringing our unconscious self into consciousness. It can also correct impressions that were formed from belief systems that no longer work in our life.

The second period of our sojourn as a human on Earth is a significant time. Within this period are many answers. Answers will be searched for, tested, accepted and denied. Choices will be made and paths will be designed. All of this will be done on a physical basis, a totally unconscious basis, a subconscious basis and on a conscious basis. In all ways the mind is seeing, hearing, thinking and choosing. The body is developing at a rapid pace, changing from the softness of infancy to the roundness of childhood, and the thinness of the beginning of puberty. Another period has begun! Celebrate!

LAW OF SEVENS: **Third Period**

From Childhood to Adulthood, Establishing an Identity

The third period of life begins on the fifteenth birthday and extends to the end of the twenty-first year. This is the period of puberty, the changing from childhood to adulthood. It is a time of completion of the physical cycle of growth and the development of expanding intellectual growth. The third period of life is a time of confusion and illusion. This period is the time of establishing an identity. *It is a time of learning who you are and how you fit into the world you see as yours.* It is a time of breaking away from parents and beginning to see life on your own terms, which defines *you to you.* It is also a time of reliance on beliefs and of building from beliefs as you create your own beliefs. It is the time when an illusion can direct you down a challenging path, which you may not recognize until many years later.

In this period your imagination designs what you want your physical world to become. Many times this perception is based on a false belief. Your choice may be formulated more from what you don't want to be, than what you truly want to be. This is only part of the confusion. The Soul memories are buried on a conscious basis for many Souls in this period. They have become overwhelmed by other stimuli, which carry their own lessons of the physical world. Established and acceptable beliefs have become this Soul's reality.

The growing teenager finds himself feeling very alone and without true direction. The conscious Soul knows that through the years the unconscious self, the Spirit self has slid further and further away into the darkness. It also knows that the subconscious self and the Soul memories have become buried under the rubble of life. This is the time when the ego is developing and begins to assume control of the physical reality. Suddenly, our teenager finds himself operating in the physical world only on a conscious basis. That consciousness is being controlled by a force that is strange and unfamiliar. The path the individual chooses will depend on past teachings and the strength of the belief system. Will the ego and intellect rule and the emotional part of the self disappear?

The emotional, feeling part of the self comes from the Spirit of the Soul. It comes from the heart. *True emotional growth is Spiritual development.* Spiritual growth is the growth of the heart, the life force of the physical body and the thinking mind. Each Soul is seeking balance of body, mind and Spirit. We enter each new life as a Spirit joining with the human element of the physical. We use the first two periods of life developing the body and the mind to the level of our Spirit. In the third period our body and mind have developed to the point of overwhelming control of the Spirit, and we are again out of balance, but not for long.

We enter each incarnation as a Spirit Consciousness. To learn our lessons completely, we must maintain our balance of body, mind and Spirit. We are one in the human form. As we progress in the Law of Sevens, we find our body has been created and our thinking mind is in the process of development. But the societal attachment to our belief system has allowed the Spirit to become overshadowed. At this time in our evolution, the function of the body is being controlled by the intellectual and egotistical part of the thinking mind. The energy balance of self is assuming a lopsided appearance. If you have a flat tire on your car at 60 miles per hour, you can feel the lopsided energy of your tires as you try to stop the car. It is hard to keep the car on the road as you try to slow down. When we find our energy unbalanced, we find it hard to stay on our chosen path of life, which creates the "wobble effect" in the thinking mind.

The Three Parts of the Mind

The mind consists of three parts: The rational mind, the intellectual mind and the intuitive mind. The rational mind is the logical part of our thinking mind that draws from all of our past learning. You look at a problem and the memory of past experience puts all aspects of the problem together. This is the "Soul" of the mind that is functioning all together. The intellectual part of the mind is the part controlled primarily by the ego. It is the part that responds to beliefs and teachings by learning the relationship of self to information. It is the storage bank for data. It collects information. It is self-focused. It operates totally from the physical consciousness level. The intuitive mind provides sensing and feeling in the thinking process. It is our "gut sense," and it functions from the Spiritual senses rather than the physical (Earth) senses. It is the unexplained knowing that we many times feel. It is a sixth sense. A psychic sense. The intuitive mind is the "Spirit" of the thinking mind.

During the third period of life, these three parts of our mind are constantly integrating and searching. They are testing each other for supremacy. But they are testing in the physical world, with the energy of the physical world as their influence. The career we choose is many times indicative of which part of the mind won in its battle for control. In this instance, as in all instances, the ideal is to remain open-minded and use each component of the thinking mind equally. Anyone who focuses only on the perceptions of the intellect is focusing on the ego self and is denying the other parts of the mind and the relationship that he or she has to the world around them. He is losing sight of the Universe and his eternal relationship with the Universe. He is placing himself totally out of balance as he envisions himself as the "I" of life. He is becoming physical matter with an intellectual mind. He is becoming "computer" controlled. He is becoming an ego robot within the physical world. We learn to become controlled by a small part of our thinking mind that works very much like a computer. This happened aeons ago when we were first created as humans.

When any human focuses totally on the intellectual self, he/she is functioning primarily with a physical focus and using only minimal considerations for the rational aspects of self. This is the primary way that we deny the world around us, including all of the other human beings. We can never deny the world that we live in. We adapt memory energy to the physical reality of our world without consciously understanding the source of the memory, because we believe that we live only one physical life. How can we not be out of balance and confused when we know so very little about ourselves?

When we focus totally on the intuitive aspects of the thinking mind, the focus is primarily in the Spiritual concepts of life as we understand them from a physical perspective and we will again remove ourselves from the world of thinking primarily from the physical reality. We will not find attunement in confusion or denial. We may be different than our peers. We will withdraw from other people because of the difference that we feel within ourselves, but we will not find balance until we reach the point of truly understanding ourselves as a physical person being guided by Spirit Consciousness.

The mind is the Universal bridge to the human body and Spirit. Part of the mind functions on a physical level and part of the mind functions on the Dual Soul level. At the Spiritual level, both parts of the mind will be acted out in the physical reality. Therefore, there must be a body-mind coordination and a mind-Spirit coordination to achieve the integrated whole, or the balance of the mind self in human form, as different parts of our human self learn how to function together as one to support us as human beings. *When we live life after life and see ourselves as simply physical beings, we miss the point of being human.* Our reality is a conscious choice for each of us, and it is as it needs to be for the lessons we need to learn as human beings. There is no right or wrong choice in life. There are no accidents in the world. Life is a never-ending energy; only the physical reality is limited by time. In the subconscious, or Soul of self, the struggle for balance never ends. It can be compared to any form of competitive sport. At any one moment our intellect/ physical body may be in charge but in the next it may be our Spirit, a focus of the Soul, or it might be our ego. Never lose sight of the integration of us as human beings on a cellular level. The integration of all of our past life memories is inherent within each of us. It is our resistance and denial that makes it difficult for us to acknowledge the truth of self. It is our belief system that presents the opposites to the perfection of Spirit energy within all of the human species.

The choices made in this third period of life are made based on the learning, the belief system, and our perception of each of the lessons during the first two periods of our life experience. No two Souls will have the same reaction to the identical set of circumstances. The understanding during these years is influenced by our perception, our Soul memory that we are carrying with us from our past lives and the level of awareness which we have reached as a Soul of these ancient memories. Perception is based on the intellect, the ego, the belief system, the understanding, the awareness level and the Soul memory. Each of our realities is a web of trilocular-designed energies, overlapping and merging to create the next design. The development of the Soul memory in the physical world changes our perception of all behaviors and actions. These memories primarily have to do with past lessons learned by the Dual Soul. Soul memory will prevent the absorption of our belief system and is another indication of an old Soul on Earth. Old Souls do not need the support of societal beliefs. They are more *comfortable* standing alone. They do not view the world as a place of competition with their immediate contemporaries, but rather as a classroom for the development and growth of their own Dual Soul.

We all participate in life to learn lessons, but we participate on a dynamically different vibratory level of energy which is unique to each of us. The vibratory energy level is determined by the intention for involvement, which will come from the level of energy that we are living. What we already understand influences our reaction to each and every physical happening. Growth is always true on a physical level just as it is true on a Dual Soul memory level and a Spirit memory level when we consciously work with our thinking mind to remember and to expand our understanding. Lessons learned do not have to be relearned in the Spirit world. It is only on Earth that we create illusion which requires relearning, to allow true learning. In the Spirit world there is only love, truth, and perfection. There are no physical illusions in the Spirit world.

"Karma" and Learning our Primary Lesson

All lessons that we truly learn become instant Spirit memory. But in the physical sense, "learned" is the key word in this statement. Many lessons that we consider to be "learned" are just a momentary awareness that in itself becomes lost with rebirth and our participation in a new life. This is why we see ourselves as continuing to make the same mistakes over and over in a physical lifetime. If we fail to truly learn, we will bring that lesson back with us into the next and the next incarnation until the lesson is learned by a complete understanding. A lesson that continues to return with each incarnation is identified in our world as "Karma." Karma is Dual Soul repetition.

Spirit memory is reflected in the function of the intuitive mind. This is in no way connected to the function of the intellect. Intellect and ego require scientific support of all information. Intuition requires faith and trust in the "Spirit self," which is our ancient memory. Intellect and ego usually find faith and trust untrustworthy. Our intellect usually defines people as functioning from faith and trust with a variety of names which most people are familiar with, such as "Saintly" or religious. Those Souls are still at a primary level of searching, because they do not understand Energy and what it means to us as human beings. As a human population we have many lessons to learn on Earth, but learning the truth of ourselves as eternal energy beings is the primary lesson.

When a Soul incarnates to the Earth plane, it comes to Earth with a Spiritual prospectus. It has total awareness at that moment of all the lessons that it wants to learn. A plan has been formulated with other Souls that outlines the various paths that can be chosen for this to be accomplished. The other Souls that have agreed to help with this learning process are identified. We choose our parents, our siblings, some of our other relatives, the people we will meet in life, those we will marry. At that moment we know what our course is, in a loose format. Along with this knowing, we are given the free will of choice, which will be used throughout our physical lifetime.

As you become involved in life, and the Law of Action and Reaction, events will occur in relationship to the Spiritual design that you have created for yourself. The reactions then are determined, not by the Spiritual prospectus, but by the belief system that you have absorbed as a physical human being and how you react to your own belief system. This would not hold true if life were predetermined, but no one's life is ever predetermined except by each human being in relationship to the lessons that are not yet learned. Only lessons are predetermined. How we eventually learn our lessons depends on our perception, the Soul memories, our awareness, and our actions and reactions to the influences in this physical existence. There is no right or wrong. Life simply IS.

In this third level we set the stage for our next life drama. We set the stage and put the props into place and the actors of our life appear on our stage. The actions that we set into motion determine the reaction in the drama of our life. That action has been molded by the beliefs that we have accepted as real and valid to us in our individual world of growth and change. Leaders are not afraid to choose by personal choice, rather than group influence. But if you learn to depend on the group influence at this point in your development, it will in itself help to mold the reality that you create as life because it will allow you to learn and change at a more rapid pace by the interaction that you have with other people. It takes intense Soul involvement to have the courage to be different in your world. It takes faith, trust, and personal strength. It takes an intuitive knowing that you can do anything you want to do, if you truly want to do it and if you understand the structure of what you want to do. This is the period to start developing the traits that you want to live in your life to *become you.* In this development there will always be the fluidity of movement and change. This is a part of the interaction of our life events. *What you are, how you live, and how you think will influence what you will be.* At any given time in your life, you will be unconsciously influencing the person that you become in later life. You will be creating *you* through the most perfect knowledge that you are willing to put into your thinking mind. There are truly no accidents within the Universe because as human beings we are always challenging ourselves.

Always, along our path, there will be choices that can bring dramatic change. The best choice is not always chosen. Many times this happens because of the fear of being different, of being true to the intuitive self. This fear is frequently found in this particular period of early development. This is the fear of separation that enters into our life consciously, for perhaps the first time. The drama of life as it reaches a crescendo is like the music of an opera as it rises and falls, seeks its own rhythm, vibrates to its own resonance, changes and flows, moving in and out through the fabric of sound. You are pure energy. Sound is pure energy. Light is pure energy. You are living the drama of life as your energy. It is beautiful, creative, motivating, and satisfying all at once. It is the you of your energy essence, on the physical plane. It is development, growth, learning and living.

This third stage is literally writing the music for the fourth stage of the Law of Sevens. Part of the music is the fulfillment of your physical development. Physical development starts music that plays another tune, which may or may not be in harmony with your intellectual development. Physical development seeks physical gratification, as part of the reality of Nature. This brings the energy of the physical senses into full bloom and lights the fires of creation.

Some people will accept this energy surge at the physical level, and actually start the act of physical creation. Others will indulge in the emotion of romantic love, allowing their feelings to lead them into physical creation. Some will walk softly through this sea of emotional energy and physical explosions, staying intact in their intellectual energy and beliefs. The paths are many, as many as there are Souls to create. Nothing is wrong. It simply IS. The IS, is your creation of your own personal physical reality. There is always the joy in the creation of the moment; whether or not it remains a joy for an entire lifetime remains to be seen.

During the third period of our life, the IS is of our world. We will cling to the IS more tenaciously in this period than in any other period of our physical life. You have latched on to your belief system and you have made it your world, your IS, your creation. You have created your identity from the beliefs that you have attached yourself to. Your beliefs in what you have done are complete. You are a child in the Garden of Eden and you have eaten fruit from the "tree of knowledge." You have gained control of your identity. You know who you are.

You have changed your perception of the world. You have become an intellectual! The ego, the "I" of you, is now in full control.

At this period of your life, you find yourself feeling smarter than you will ever be again. You compare your intellect with others around you, and they suddenly seem rather simple, while you are bursting with knowledge and wisdom. This is an illusion. It is symbolic of the illusions the mind will continue to create and it is equally unreal. At that very moment, which is indeed your point of power, it is real to you and you have created that reality. As puberty passes through adolescence and into adulthood, your belief is focused on yourself. Your intellectual mind is ruling supreme. Few escape this illusion, and this is the time for it to be and to be enjoyed.

Your world goes speeding along, the drama of life being the one of beliefs. The beliefs that you have attached yourself to become your world. You will march across the country, sleep in the street, go to war, run away from home or do any number of other things to uphold those beliefs that have become your identity. Your physical growth has slowed down and you are feeling strong and healthy. Little if any concern is being given to preservation of the physical self. At this moment your beliefs are more important than you are, in your thinking mind. You are serenely following your belief system, eating as you have learned to eat, sleeping as you have learned to sleep, functioning as you have learned to function. You are engrossed in your drama of life. You feel indestructible.

This is only one more illusion, in your drama. Your cellular function is changing again and preparing your body for adulthood. It needs restoration for the cellular changes that are ahead. New challenges, new activities, new thoughts all require abundant energy. Energy of the physical self must always come from the restoration of the water, organic mineral salts, and the vitamins that the body desperately needs for cellular function. There is not a time in our physical life when this reality is not true. In this period of tremendous change it is essential to eat organic foods, drink pure water, and breathe fresh air to restore your chemical design that you know as yourself.

A body deprived of its vital nutrients will not wither and die away in a day, a month, or a year, but we will create a definite cellular drama that we may be totally unaware of happening in our physical body. At any point in time the survival of our physical body is dependent upon how we live. The choice of pure food is essential, which helps the cells of the body to adjust. If the adjustment is manifested in the way of problems that we do not recognize or that are not recognized by our world as the body's physical cravings for the Earth's nutrients, many illnesses will be created.

Some of the manifestations can be acne, nausea, emotional instability, depression, feelings of suicide, irritability, sleeplessness, unusual behavior, overeating, drug or alcohol addiction, hyperactivity, learning or motor impairment, and a variety of physical diseases such as cancer or mental illness. Many diseases are minor in our terms during this period, because the deficiencies have had only from birth to twenty-one to accumulate. For some, the deficiencies may have been present at birth because of deficiencies in the mother. The chemical deficiencies in the mother can produce what is known as genetic or congenital disease. For some the dis-ease and disease can produce a very difficult reality of slow disease expansion that will end eventually in death.

In our physical reality the deficiencies create the excesses and the excesses create the deficiencies in our body. The physical body that is in a state of true balance has no cravings. This person will not need and will not be capable of surviving on medications, drugs, alcohol, and our basically non-nutrient foods such as fats, starches, and sugars. Our life and our health must be clarified with relationship to our chemical requirements. Not all of the fats and starches are non-nutrient, but people crave poor or non-nutrient processed foods the most. Examples of this are the many junk foods, candies, desserts, and pastries that people crave which are produced from fat, refined white flour, salt and sugars. These are high calorie foods that have little if any nutrient value.

By the time that we consume many foods, they have little if any of Nature's true bounty of nutrients left. Sugar tends to decrease the appetite, and eating natural foods that will maintain the cellular viability of the physical self can keep you healthy, where "junk" foods can leave you malnourished. We may crave these foods and be capable of consuming large quantities at one sitting, but we have not consumed foods that will protect the health of our body and keep us well and active. Eating many sweet foods is equivalent in the body's chemical/ physiological response to drinking alcohol. We feel a rush of warmth and energy very quickly after consuming these high sugar products.

Unfortunately, this "high" is not one that provides the nutrients which the body needs for balance. It will soon wear off and we will again crave something to eat, or we may find ourselves severely depressed and tired. Nutritional deficiencies among the youth of this specific time period have the potential for depression and suicide. If this doesn't happen, addiction to drugs or alcohol may be the chosen path for this Soul.

In this period you will find the frankly obese and the very thin individual suffering from serious malnutrition. Each physical body has its own level of balance. This level of balance does not come from counting calories or pounds. It comes from the correct replacement of the essential nutritional elements of the Earth, which is the true basis of our cellular structure and function. During this period eating habits deteriorate and produce an imbalance within the body that leads to additional stress. Good habits of eating from Nature's food that were established early in life will prove to be invaluable in this quickly changing period. If good eating habits have not been taught before this period in life, it will be difficult to change them during these years of confusion and illusion.

The stress and confusion of this period are compounded by peer pressure, which makes it difficult to live the way we may wish to live without being different. During this period being different becomes a way of being a follower or a leader. Being different at this time is frequently seen as being different in relationship to those you see as authority figures, and in not being different from your contemporaries. So the shift here is to being a follower of your own peer group. This identification attachment will follow throughout life, unless there is a conscious decision to change the belief. In the inherent need to be different from the establishment, this group of Souls becomes a clone of fads and foolishness.

It is all part of growth and the breaking away process, which our society accepts as necessary among families. In the Universal concept this separation is the opposite of the unity that we are striving for and therefore it serves as a lesson for those who need it in this incarnation. The confusion of this period makes it difficult to focus on survival of the physical, which is the true goal of the body function. It is a testing of each and every Soul to see if they indeed desire to complete this life as planned. Incarnations are planned for the purpose and process of learning lessons as we grow from infancy to old age. If it appears to the Soul that the situation they have grown into does not allow them to learn the exact lesson which they came to learn, they may choose another lesson and continue or they may decide to leave Earth's plane.

In the time of war, there will be a collective group of Souls who are ready to return to the Spirit plane. If there is no war, they will find another way. Nothing is pre-ordained in our Earth life, except Souls are on Earth to learn lessons. Many times the patterns we create as a means of learning the lessons are very challenging for us to understand. It is always a matter of choice for the Soul, although that choice will be made from the subconscious level, not the conscious level. Parents who understand the need for good nutritional habits during the first, second and third period of life will help that child understand the internal Soul need to protect the physical temple.

Growth into the other periods of life will usually be smoother, more balanced, and therefore more consciously aware experiences for the Soul. Learning the value of protection of the body as the physical temple is a giant step forward in the evolution of the Dual Soul. It is the ideal step forward and should be created as conscientiously by the parent as the child was nourished in infancy. Balancing the physical in the infant, child, and adolescent keeps the mind and Spirit open and aware. This requires discipline, structure, guidance, teaching and most of all LOVE. Parents are caretakers, they are not owners. They must teach by example and word, not by demands.

Life does not grow well under dictatorships, just as a world, a culture, and a business do not grow well under dictatorships. Freedom and openness are virtues that are also learned as children. They will not be learned without a child's experience of love. Our progeny will eat as we eat and as we feed them. This is why diseases appear to be genetically determined. It is not so much genetics as it is the improper learning and habit of re-creation of events with the choices of food that is being eaten.

In cultures many Souls experience the same nutritional deficiencies, just as they do in sub-cultures and poor families. They also marry and produce offspring within this same cultural system, which is learned by the youth and transferred into their family situations. Therefore, the "genetic patterning" and the same diseases will be found, which supports the toxicity of the same eating habits that will also be flourishing throughout many generations of family lives.

Genetic disease is an illusion of our world. This will be understood later by our society as an early destruction of the genetic code through improper eating which will be passed on. Unfortunately, we continue to look at disease for the answer to dis-ease.

We must learn to look for the deficiencies and excesses in nutrition and lifestyle of individuals for our answers to the physical self and its diseases. Excesses and deficiencies in lifestyle affect the mind through the beliefs, the attitude, and the behavioral rhythms of the body. This passing down of behaviors and beliefs is a serious problem for many in our world. When we fail to give our body the nutrients that it needs, the body will always become sick and diseased. When our quality of food is challenged, disease is the result. Cancer is a perfect example of how we are harming ourselves with inappropriate nutrition and our inability to understand ourselves.

We always create our own personal reality, and in the physical sense, this is literal truth. We are the perfect example of body-mind coordination as we were designed to be. There is no other way. Give this child of puberty and adolescence the foods of the Earth. Let his balance be as complete as you can manage. Keep him free of waste material. *Understand that three things must occur for physical health. They are digestion, assimilation, and elimination of Nature's food.* If there is a problem with any of these three levels, the physical body will not be balanced. Without the proper foods, these three bodily functions will not happen normally as they should. Improper nutritional intake will eventually reveal a problem with one or all of these bodily functions which allows the individual to create disease.

This is true throughout life and can be used as one barometer of proper eating. In our world today this statement can be validated by the amount of money being spent on digestive aids and laxatives. Our diseases are all the result of deficiencies of nutrients and excesses that are being provided to the body and mind. One reason for this is the junk foods that are being eaten. This can also be validated by the money spent on diseases and dying. Once we can change the way that we think, we will change our behaviors that are leading us into an early death.

The ending of this period in the Law of Sevens is the turning point in the existence of the Earth sojourn for any Soul. We are ready for true independence as a human species. We are now responsible for self as an individual. We have reached adulthood. The lesson for us as parents is let your child be an adult. For the Soul involved it is accept the responsibility of and for yourself. In so doing you become a self-sufficient, functional, and healthy ADULT, and you will be totally responsible for every decision that you make regarding your personal life.

Relationship Profiles *PHYSICAL (ego) Mind Focus*	*Personality Traits* *SPIRITUAL Mind Focus*
External Perception and Interpretation of Life	Internal Perception and Interpretation of Life
Argumentative	Open to Discussion (dialogue)
Closed Mind/Fear	Open Mind/Love
Controlling	Free
Judgmental	Understanding
Non-Communicative	Open to Communication (Self-Expressive)
Unstable Thinking/Labile	Stable Thinking/Balanced
Guilt-Ridden	Comfort (able)
Fear of Life and People	Love of Self, Life and People
Separateness	Integration/Unity
Inequality	Equality
Untruth/Lying	Truth
Inadequate	Capable (creative)
Worthless	Value Self and Life
Dependent	Independent
Irresponsible	Responsible
Weakness	Strength
Anxiety/Apprehension	Power
Cowardice	Courage
Negative/Derogatory Language/Cursing	Loving Language
Violence/Combative	Gentle/Non-Combative
Self-Centered/Narcissistic	Caring and Sharing
Reclusive/Withdrawn	Vivacious

LAW OF SEVENS: **Fourth Period**

Who do you want to be?

The beginning of the fourth period of the Law of Sevens finds the Dual Soul entering into the stage of adulthood. This span covers the years twenty-one through twenty-eight. It is a time of self-realization. It is the beginning of manhood and womanhood. It is the recognition of your selfhood by the world that you know and live in. You have passed the test of growing up. You are an adult. It is the beginning of the feeling of internal power, and you have decisions that you must make that will determine the years ahead of you that you must live. Who do you want to be?

Internal power is accepted as the world of the intellect. This is your moment in time to prove that you can be responsible for you. It is the time to put your stamp on the world that you know. It is a time to stretch your wings, to sow your oats, to be you. This, too, is an illusion. You are you at the moment of birth. You develop into a larger physical you, but many times much of importance is lost along the way. Getting the body, mind and Spirit out of balance is not truly representative of us as a Spiritual Being living on Earth. That is why, amidst all of the glory, there is that feeling of frustration, of searching, of knowing that something that is essential to your well-being is missing. We are challenged to open our thinking mind to our new role of Personal Responsibility.

The Soul will remind the intellectual mind that the balance is being upset. Activity begins to escalate. Time rushes on. You have joined the fast-paced world of living and working. Suddenly the stillness is no longer there for you. It must be searched out, planned for and cherished.

As adults we continue to learn behaviors and beliefs, as we have in the first three periods of our life. Suddenly, the concept of success takes on a new image. The concept of work changes and balloons. The concept of relationships becomes molded by the world that we are seeking. We have not yet learned how to be an individual and make our own choices based on our own Dual Soul desires. We are now in the process of "branding" ourself for the world. We are in the process of saying, "I am a doctor, lawyer, Indian Chief." We are putting ourselves in a category that will take us a lifetime to overcome.

You have not been able to control the ego. You feel the need to belong. You do not yet understand that you are you but you remain a part of the human race. You are not willing to go out on a limb and identify yourself as "I AM ME." This would be a total break with the needs and practices of our society. You have been taught to conform. You have been taught to identify with "something," as a completion of your own identity. In the Universe you are perfect, just the way you are. Your identity of self, as a Soul, needs no physical identifiers. What you do with your life, what you become in life, depends totally and completely upon the way that you relate to the mind of self within as how you think.

Success is Knowing Thyself

Graduating from Yale does not make you a good person. It does not make you a success in life. It does not make you happy. It makes you a graduate of Yale. Leaders do not conform. They are at peace within. They will participate in the activities of the world but inside they will know themselves. They will follow their own inner voice and they will follow it in total peace and joy. It will matter what they do. That, too, will be accepted as one more step in the evolution of their Soul. They will work with humility and joy. Their physical identity is connected to the Soul, not to a physical association. They understand their ability to be successful because that is what they are patterned to do in life. They have peace and joy in the pursuit of their work, play, and everyday BEING in life.

Followers will conform, internally and externally. They will live the belief of the "need of association for identity." They will not feel comfortable without that association to complete the mental picture that they have painted for themselves from our cultural system. They will sincerely believe that they cannot be successful or happy unless they have fulfilled their image of self as having graduated from "Yale," having become a "lawyer," living in the "right house," in the "right part of town," and married to the "perfect spouse," etc. Their belief is not in their own perfection and capability, it is in the "props" of their belief system that they have become attached to and will live by in multiple lives until they learn enough to grow beyond their beliefs.

The Earth is a mass of followers. Our recognized leaders are true followers. They, more than the average person, are following the structured belief system of our society. Being a true leader is being true to the Spirit Self. Only we know if we are being true to that Higher Energy of ourselves within as our personal guide. This knowing will be subconscious but it will be reacted to on a conscious level. If you live in a state of inner peace and consistent joy, you are on the right path. Being true to self gives you that peace and joy. You feel instinctively good and happy. You appreciate the sun, moon, sea and Earth around you. You breathe the air and rejoice in the living. Your work is an expression of your love of life and you are love only as you live it. You are in tune with the feeling-tones of Nature. You are Nature. In this image you see yourself as complete and successful.

Intellectual Development: The Building of an Open Mind

The fourth period is a period of intellectual development and building of the mind. The two are not the same. Intellectual development is just that – it is developing the intellect and accumulating knowledge. It is the gathering and storing of information. This is essential in our development and it is the basis for mind integration. Building the mind is, in the Universal sense, building the three parts of the mind, the rational mind, the intellectual mind, and the intuitive mind. This requires that we first and foremost have an open mind. Maintaining an open mind, in all parts of the mind, is contrary to the belief system of our world. Because of the denial that exists in our society, open-mindedness challenges you to be you.

The intellect should not be in total control of any human life. But it can be used in the total development of the mind. *Intelligence is the ability to learn with feeling.* This is not confined to one aspect of information, but rather it is an indication of openness to the lifelong process of human growth. This is processing the facts of life through our heart as well as through our head. Intelligence means that we do not believe everything we hear simply because we heard it. Intelligence is the connection that exists between our heart and our mind.

There must be a balance. We must be open to Soul memories, to learning and to sensing. We must be able to assimilate information with feeling. This period is the return to conscious awareness for all of us as human beings. It is a crucial period for Soul growth, and it is essential to our evolution as a Spirit Consciousness. In our physical world this is also the period of creation. This is the period of our physical lives that is devoted to creating relationships and children. It is a time for creating homes and careers. It is also a time to create and discover the real you. We can see the real "us" when we learn to use the rational mind. The rational mind knows that we cannot be happy and productive if we are not in association with other people, not active in the stream of life, and not expanding our mind with new thought. This is why marriage is a healing for many people on Earth.

If during your formative years from birth to now, you have expanded your awareness of your true relationship to the Universe, you will be consciously operating with more than your five senses. You will consciously be building your body and your mind, with the positive Universal approach to your reality. You will know that you are creating your own reality. You will accept the responsibility for your actions and reactions as your reality begins to take form and have meaning. You will understand that living cannot be productive for you when your thoughts are based in another person's belief system. You will understand those moments in your world that work for you and those that work against you. If you are working within a belief system and awareness enters into your thinking mind, you will begin the changes that are necessary to sustain your own creation. You may find yourself examining your beliefs and your actions. You may know intuitively that changes are in order. You may not know immediately what changes to make. This is of little concern. *Knowing the precise path is not as important as the recognition that there is an alternative path for you.* You can choose alternatives with time and in peace as the alternate paths begin to appear for you. The paths are always there. When you resist them, deny them, fail to understand them, they will not be perceived in relationship to you and your growth.

This is the time when we seek to know concepts that have been unknown to us until this moment in our lives. Recognition of alternatives, in this period, will protect you from becoming closed and protective with your inner self. You will not function from fear, but rather from the love of self and the love of others. This will create a positive reality in which to grow and share. The fears that have come with you from childhood usually gain strength in this period of your life.

The newness of total individual responsibility for yourself opens you to hidden insecurities. You become vulnerable to the hidden fears and anxieties of your childhood. These anxieties will encourage you to become more attached to the belief system that has supported you in your early life. You may comply with these beliefs even though you may feel uncomfortable deep down inside of your mind.

For many Souls who have grown up in organized religion, believing in guilt, sin, and punishment, pain and disease become their concept of life and will design their death. Guilt, sin, and punishment are human creations, not Spirit creations. They function because the belief that they exist creates the reaction within our human life as we evolve. Souls that are in negative energy, attached to negative belief systems, will continue to attract negative energy. They will find themselves in bad marriages, unfulfilling jobs, destructive relationships, and friendships that do not last. They will be continuously fighting dis-ease and disease. The mind is the builder of our physical world as well as our physical body.

When you find yourself in negative energy, acknowledge it and change it. The mind is more capable of building the positive energy because the Universal energy is positive, the Spiritual energy is positive, and the Earth energy is positive. Working within the framework of the positive energy forces provides less resistance to positive creation. All of us will find ourselves working hard to create some of our negativity and drama. A mind that must build with negative concepts is building from the unknown, and the unlearned. We are the light of love and truth, in the beginning. That is our true Soul memory, and it is present at all times in our evolution. It is perhaps the easiest energy for the mind to remember from past lives, and it is also the easiest energy for the negative mind to resist.

At birth we are perfection. Our Soul remains perfect. Our body and mind are subject to all physical human dramas, whether they are positive or negative influences. During this period, the development of awareness will alter the aging process. Negative thoughts will be fewer. We will understand our body's relationship to Nature more. When these two concepts exist in conjunction with each other you will be doing everything you can do to improve your physical body and you will do very little to destroy it. Life will usually look extremely good at this period of our evolution as human beings.

When we can recognize that we are part of Nature, and we can also recognize our dependency on the elements of Nature for our physical existence, we are growing in our thought process and our evolution is showing us how it works to assist us in our changes and health. We have acknowledged the dependency of our physical body on air and water. We understand that the oxygen we breathe is in the exact proportion that allows all humans to thrive on Earth. Spirit made it perfect for our life as a human being. Air is the Universal purifier but we have added the pollution that makes our air toxic. Toxic sprays are used in the home today and are the cause of several diseases. We admit to the need for water, but we still do not yet realize that toxic water makes our body toxic and pure water adds to the health and happiness of our body. The more comfortable we are with the constant use of water both internally and externally, the more we appreciate its value in our lives. Water does more than most of the medicine that we use. Water is the universal purifier therefore it is the universal medicine, when it is pure. Water has total healing power. When we drink pure water in the amount that our body needs, we always support our body's health. Most water is polluted because we have polluted our land.

Water is the second element that Spirit established as essential to the function of the physical body. Our physical body is primarily water. Water is the internal balancing element for total cellular function and health. Should the physical body be in a state of imbalance, the most efficient method of returning it to total balance is by drinking water. In our world today, physicians do this with intravenous fluids. If we can drink, we can balance our body fluids. Soaking in a tub of warm water will have some effect, but drinking will be more efficient for the total body with no trauma and its effect is quicker. If the water level within the body is inadequate, the body will work as a sponge when placed in water, which is also important.

Water was the first medicine and medical therapy used by the human being. It is still the best overall therapy. Our culture will reach a point in its evolution when this will be accepted and practiced. Water treats the whole person, the whole body, the mind and the Spirit. It literally takes the stress away from the body, mind, and Spirit with its soothing influence. Water is equivalent to the hand of Spirit soothing our body and mind. Yet most of us, including the medical community, do not have the proper appreciation for water.

The recognition of the other elements of Nature necessary for the perfect function of our body has been misunderstood, misdirected, and ignored. We are made from Earth, are of the Earth and must replenish the balance of our cellular design from the Earth. For us to live vitally, our body must be replenished with these vital mineral elements of Earth to assure total viability of cellular structure and function. These elements of the soil are found in the foods of Nature. No other foods or drugs are assimilated as efficiently by the body. In 1948 when our government and the chemical industry began creating chemicals for the soil, we also created the pattern of diseases, especially cancer, which we are continuing to attempt to understand. The primary disease created from chemicals being put on the soil was and is cancer, which is expanding each year.

All of us are now living with a false sense of security, especially regarding our health. When we live with the opinion that we can eat whatever we may choose from de-vitaminized, de-mineralized and man-made chemically polluted foods and replace these elements with man-made vitamins and minerals within our body, we are living a fatal illusion. During the period of the first, second and third Law of Sevens, our food may have been prepared for us from contaminated sources. We may not have had an awareness of the value of pure and natural foods from Nature at any time in our physical lives. If the eating habits that we were taught concentrated on fast foods, processed foods, prepared foods, high fat and sugar foods, now is the time for change.

We are now adults and totally responsible for our own habits and beliefs. Life is about change! In changing the foods that we eat to organic foods, we become happier and healthier people and we can live happier and longer lives. We can successfully restore and cleanse our body at any time in our life, if our mind and our body are in complete coordination. This includes cleansing the body of disease. It does not matter what damage has been done with previous eating habits if we are at least fairly healthy. We now have the opportunity to change. We can make a conscious decision to be well and healthy. If we are living a period of primarily minor physical annoyances, we are living the groundwork that has been laid for more serious physical problems that can erupt into disease.

The beginning of adulthood is the perfect time to stop and evaluate all of our belief systems, especially those related to eating. While you are deciding who you are from the intellectual sense, also decide who you are from the physical sense and who you are from the emotional sense. You are a trilocular whole and no part of your self stands alone on Earth. The body, mind, and Spirit that is you works in unison. If your mind is confused, your body and Spirit are confused. If your body is sick, your mind and Spirit are sick. If your Spirit has been denied, your mind and body have been denied.

Direct your growth in all three areas of self just as you plan to direct your career for total growth. We can never be singular so we should never focus on a single aspect of self. Having a single focus builds a fence around you. It shuts you off from family, friends, and the world. It destroys relationships. The body, mind, and Spirit are constantly striving to become more of an integrated whole, as we evolve in Earth evolution and Soul evolution. The awareness of this internal intention can help you with your individual progress. It will help you with your everyday problems of life.

Each lesson that we learn becomes a vital part of our Soul memory. Each lesson that we fail to learn becomes Karma, or repetition, for the next life experience or incarnation. We control our progress by our conscious awareness of what each moment of our physical life is teaching us. Evaluation and focus at this point in our life will be an advantage to our growth. The NOW is our point of power. Seek the fresh foods from the Earth. These are vegetables, fruits, nuts, seeds and grains. They easily provide the necessary elements of Nature that most of us are deficient in and will protect us from aging and disease.

Contrary to many belief systems, we can obtain all of the protein, vitamins, and minerals that our physical body demands for cellular function from the Earth. More important for us, we will remove the excesses from our diet that produce waste material and blockage within our physical body if we will eat of these first generation foods. Our diet and lifestyle raise our nutrient requirements to the level we now believe it to be. An example of this problem is calcium. We know that digestion, assimilation and elimination are required to maintain a healthy body.

Calcium and other nutrients are only digested and assimilated when the foods are primarily Nature's foods and we are living a natural life. Calcium absorption is not complete if we eat too much meat, ingest too many chemicals (including medicines and food preservatives), drink too much alcohol, or do not exercise in the proper amount. Therefore, the proper perception of this problem is not that we do not eat enough calcium, but rather that we eat too much meat, drink too much alcohol, ingest too many chemicals, and do not exercise enough.

Eating animal meats is harmful because of the present feeding system of the animals and the fat and chemicals that they present to the human body. Some meats have less fat than others and can be of value because of their protein. Enjoying meats in small amounts will be beneficial to the body if the natural foods are continued, too. The problem occurs when the diet is primarily meat. When you have a diet with an excess of protein and fat, you will not be eating fiber and natural elements. Meat has some fiber, but it does not contain many of the essential food elements, although it is high in protein. If our mind craves meat, wild game is an alternative that has less fat to pollute the body. The waste products from meat do accumulate and do cause disease in our culture. In small amounts meat will help with the cellular structure, if it can be obtained in a close to natural state.

This seven-year period is a period of rejuvenation and change. Our entire world has changed. Our concept of self has changed. Our responsibility has changed. Best of all, these aspects of change are all within our control. There is no one to blame for our actions but us. We have accepted the responsibility for self. Never, for the rest of our life, forget that we are creating our own reality. When we create our own reality, we are always responsible for what we create.

If the physical reality that you are in is not happy and joyful, change the reality or your perception of that reality. It is possible to initiate internal and external change that will bring you joy and happiness within nearly any situation. If you find change within a situation impossible for you, then you may find that leaving a job, a relationship, an environment or whatever, is the appropriate choice. Under these circumstances, it will be necessary to look internally for your lesson or you will repeat the same situation with your next activity. Our Soul grows and changes by the very act of living our Soul lessons. If we fear the very concept of living lessons, we are afraid of life on a very deep level, which we may need to explore.

The fourth period of the Law of Sevens is the beginning of the development of awareness for us. We have been living with very little concept of why we are living our human life. Many people do not think twice about what it means to live our life. Life is about our growth. As we live, we do grow and change even when we feel we would like for change not to happen. The more we resist life the more we resist growth. As human beings, we are designed to grow and change. Our changes may be subtle. Caring for the health of our body, mind, and Spirit is a true joy. It will allow us the most in Soul evolution for the next period of the Law of Sevens.

LAW OF SEVENS: **Fifth Period**

During the years between twenty-nine and thirty-five, we are living the fifth period of our life. This is an important period in the development cycle of Earth's existence for all human beings. During this period we truly set the beliefs of our world into action. We feel the searching that occurred in the fourth period less intensely. We begin to "feel" that we know who we are and what we want. Can we design what we want and make it happen in our lives through our clever design? We live in a fairytale world, which determines how we think about our life and its relationship to us. What are we doing? What do we want to do? What do we want to create with our "doing"?

The true development of your world begins to take form. The form your world takes depends upon the belief system that your ego and intellect have become attached to thus far in life. In your family you can have many siblings in the same house with the same exposure to the same beliefs. These siblings will be totally different in their life direction and their Soul needs. This difference is the result of Soul awareness and the lessons that you have incarnated to learn in this lifetime. Your perception of the family, friends, and yourself will be focused by the design that you have created for your life before your incarnation, and your accomplishments may be very different than anyone else that you know. Many beliefs will materialize in many directions. Our awareness influences our understanding. Our perception of each and every single happening differs depending on the belief system and the teachings that are transmitted to the mind. Our mind takes the perception, the awareness, and the Soul memories and balances them out into our understanding of our life.

The awareness level of the Soul is determined by the level of the Soul to some degree and also the individual lessons the Soul is here to learn in this lifetime. Soul growth improves with each lesson learned; therefore our actions will reflect the purpose of the Dual Soul. This may not be immediately reflected in the physical self because the physical self is a consistent lesson of Earth incarnations. *The physical self is our method of self-instruction.* It is through the act of being physical that we can experience and learn. If we had truly learned all of our lessons, we would no longer need the physical experience. There is no other way. Our physical life is about learning and growth.

Awareness is not something static in our world. It is a fluid sense of knowing self. It is an internal sensing of the origin of self and the mission of self as life. It is a river of the mind that runs constantly with thought. As new awareness is gained the river swells and flows, only to again search for the peace of a calm balance. Our understanding is greater in quality and quantity because of the new awareness within our thinking mind. Each and every insight that increases the awareness increases the level of the river of understanding. This mind expansion creates a river of energy. Awareness is energy, knowledge is energy, and the physical matter of our bodies is energy. We are energy. *As we increase any part of self, we increase the energy of BEING.* On Earth we could be compared to a light bulb. In the beginning of life, we have a certain energy generation. We may start life comparable to a twenty-five watt bulb. When our life is ended on Earth, this energy that we have collected may change our electrical voltage to a two-hundred-watt bulb or higher. Our human energy has a magnetic quality. What we are determines what we attract. If we are positive, we will attract positive energy. If we are negative, we will attract negative energy. Have you ever known anyone that seems to have one bad happening after the other in their life? This is a person that is attracting negative energy. This does not mean that it is wrong to attract negative energy. There are lessons of life that can only be learned when we are willing to risk the attraction of negative energy. These circumstances, events or happenings are not seen as energy. These circumstances, events or happenings are not in themselves negative. They are the creation of an image that allows us to view our perception of life. It was our choice to create the image.

In this fifth period of life we are developing our world. Everything about us is in some stage of development. We will not be the same person that we were ten years ago or even five years ago. We are becoming. We are developing. We are processing and developing based on the combination of stimuli, information, and awareness that we have thus far experienced. Our belief system plays an important part in this period of life. We attach ourselves to the beliefs that work for us through the years. Now we have a map of beliefs, knowledge, Soul memories and awareness to start molding ourselves into who we want to be.

Of all the parts of the mind – the rational, intellectual, intuitive, and ego mind – that we are now functioning with, the intuitive is the hardest to acknowledge at this point in life. The learning of the belief system, which this Soul has chosen to subscribe to, has the strongest hold. The belief system creates the structure of the ego. The ego cannot allow the intuitive mind to function. During this period the ego controls most of what we understand about our reality. That too is a learning process and has its place in our life. It can be used to our advantage if our awareness level is developing adequately.

It is during this period that we begin to think and plan for retirement. We start our downhill slide physically and mentally, on an unconscious basis. We set this process in motion with our mind, by our thoughts and our actions. Our thoughts are living energy. They create unconsciously as easily as they do consciously. As we project our vision into our future, we begin to imagine ourselves in old age. Our fear inspires our physical action to provide for our future life that is in our thoughts. We look for a job that has retirement advantages. We start a retirement fund. We plan our financial world around our retirement vision. We begin to live our life in the imaginary world of Retirement, which we use to begin thinking old. We begin to lose our willingness to change. We are beginning to create an imaginary world that is out there in the future nearly thirty years away, and it becomes our reality of today. Our thoughts turn to the specific image of the future that we have created, which means that we will have difficulty creating in the reality of the present moment. We will be building what we imagine as our "future."

As we become locked into such a structured belief system, we create a habit of living in a fear of death. We stop being spontaneous. We become regimented. We stop doing the things that we enjoy. We will postpone events, waiting until we can retire. Our life and many of the things which we dream about doing are in reality put on "hold," and we continue living our fear illusions. We are saving for tomorrow. Our money lives in the bank. Our body starts to deteriorate. We sit and we watch television. We stop the activity that keeps our mind and body functioning, which allows the food that we eat to be poorly digested and absorbed, and we begin to create many diseases.

Fear takes over. Worry becomes the emotion of the day. For many of us, this worry is focused on the fear of separation from our retirement or our separation from tomorrow's job. It is a fear of being separated from the future as we have planned it that throws us off our track of living. Retirement is viewed in the imagination as the time in our life when we can be free. We imagine that we will at that magic moment be free of working, free of children, free of responsibility, free of debt, and ready to have fun. This is our most interesting illusion. Living in the vacuum of the future makes us terrified that we will never be able, indeed never live long enough to enjoy our retirement. This illusion can become overwhelming. This illusion is building a high wall around our sense of Well-Being. It is blocking out the freedom and openness of living. It creates an obsessive need to work and to save. As the time for retirement draws near, realization sets in for us that we are not the same person we were thirty years ago. Our body aches. We have huge doctor bills. The money hasn't increased as we thought it would. The reality of today is that tennis sounds too strenuous. If we sell our house and move we will have to have a new mortgage. A new mortgage means we have to work.

The illusion of an easy life begins to crumble and we lose hope. *Hope in our world is our Spirit Energy – the motivation of life. Without Spirit (hope) there is no freedom in life.* Locking ourselves into the concept of "mental and emotional imprisonment" at any moment of our life is a disadvantage. We are born as humans to enjoy change. We must be willing to live with spontaneity. We should live with joy, hope, and action every moment of our lives.

If there is no joy in what we are doing, why are we doing it?

Life is to be lived with joy in each moment that you live. There is no tomorrow. There is only today, because that is what you are focused upon. If your life does not offer you the joy and happiness that you deserve, on a day to day basis, something is out of balance in what you are doing with your life. Do not look at the rest of the world and judge it. The rest of the world is not responsible for where you are in your life. Look within yourself. Look inside, to see if you are constantly learning and expanding your mind. Do you truly know you? You have created what you have. If what you have created is making you unhappy and is not what you want, you must evaluate your life and risk the change that is necessary. Our point of power is in the present. If we fear change, we will be stuck exactly where we are, which is how decay and disease sets itself into our life. There is no other way.

Subconsciously, this imbalance, this fear, sets up a reaction of frustration within us (the self). This frustration is the recognition of the imbalance presented to the Dual Soul. The Soul recognizes only today. It deals with creating the reality of the moment, the life force of the moment. The Soul cannot deal in the reality of a future, because that is not what it is living. Within the Spirit and Soul there is no concept of time. Time, as we view it, is a created function of our ego, which allows us to divide up our time. There is only now – this precise moment. The

Spirit does not recognize physical time or space. The Spirit is infinite. The Soul is dealing with the eternity of Spirit self not the eternity of the physical body. Sending the Spirit messages of the future from the physical plane is sending it messages of now on the Spirit plane.

We live in fear of mistakes and failures. There are no mistakes and failures. There is only living and learning. The living experiences contribute to our growth. Without the willingness to change and to live, we do not experience and we do not grow. Living for retirement, or a future tomorrow, is an instant message of aging. If we must think of retirement, think of it in the now of youth. But remember that retirement itself is an illusion. It is a futuristic word in our language. Since there is only now, there is no future, no tomorrow until it happens and then it becomes today.

In this state of frustrated imbalance the body begins to be uncomfortable. It feels the change. It mentally, knowingly has not sought change. In fact, the physical self is in the belief of power. Mixed messages are many at this time in life for the physical self and the Spiritual self. The thinking mind is the liaison energy that is working with the physical and the Spiritual self. The mind, in its creative sense, is spinning off in several directions at one time with little focus on the reality of today. The mind as the builder is in the process of building. Developing an awareness of the actions and reactions of the mind is a tremendous understanding for us to grasp. At this moment in our time, understanding the power of thought is one of the many lessons that the human is trying to learn. *Understanding is learning to change negative energy to positive energy within the mind.* We do not recognize the negative effects that we have upon our body when we live in other than the present moment of our time as our power. We do not recognize that when we think we cannot see, we will begin to experience problems with our vision. Our concept of "not seeing" is our failure to understand.

The body and mind are coordinated on a literal level. When the mind fails to see, the body fails to see. As we age we become more aware of our failure to understand. This failure to understand, to see, increases our eye problems. Some problems can occur because we are working on the lesson of understanding. If the Karma of "not seeing" is a critical issue for the Soul, that Soul will choose blindness. That Soul will try to learn to "see" through the use of the other physical senses. How many times a day do you say aloud, "I cannot see" in answer to a question? Understanding the coordination between the mind and the body will encourage you to change your response to "I want to see." This is exchanging a positive statement for a negative statement. Within our body we strengthen our eyes if we introduce positive energy into the eye rather than negative energy.

Our human body is built and rebuilt moment by moment with the energy that the mind sends to it. The mind building the body is a literal physical response to our thoughts. All human exposure to our thoughts is a message to self. All human experience is a lesson within itself. Watching a war movie is producing the reality of war within us. Thoughts are real actions in the sense of energy. When "enough" of any type of energy exists on a physical level it presents a physical response. The current belief in catastrophic events, for example, will bring about catastrophic events. A belief in war will produce war. A belief that your boss is always angry will produce the perception to you that he is always angry. Your response to these events will be your response to the level of your belief.

We are continually creating our reality in direct response to our beliefs. Thoughts are things, in our physical reality as they are in all realities. They are energy. If your thoughts are negative, the energy you are attracting is negative. If your thoughts are positive, the energy you are attracting is positive. If your perception of the world is that everyone is out to "get" you, it will appear to happen that way for you. If you are driving down the street mad, be careful because you are inviting an accident. If you are living your life in an angry way, be careful because you are inviting disasters to appear in your life. Happiness and joy create the best energy for you to "light up your life." Our energy attracts energy of like quality. Our Universe is one of energy, total energy, and nothing escapes that reality. The energy of one joins with the energy of the masses to become a moving force in world events. The mind is the builder in every respect, whether it is negative or positive action. Our thoughts create our life and the world around us. All of this happens on a very dynamic level, which is perhaps confusing for us to understand in the linear concept of time and space in which our physical world exists. Leaving your mind open, without resistance, while reading this book will allow your awareness to become conscious of the energy in which you exist.

The feeling that we have during this fifth period of the Law of Sevens is one of running in circles, never having enough time, never doing all we want to do. This concept of our world as frantic confusion can give us a boost in the wrong direction in understanding what the Soul consciousness is feeling and the energy that it is sending out to the Universe. This is the development cycle in full swing. Exterior events are being precipitated by the events of the mind. Everything is happening. Life events are bursting all around us. We are responding to the activity of the developing mind.

At times a Soul comes to Earth that is reluctant to participate in all of this fragmented mind activity. The Soul may feel like secluding itself and letting the awareness develop on a different level. These Souls will manifest an obvious difference in the development of the intellectual mind. These Souls will not be what we would consider in the mainstream of life. The stream they are in can follow many paths but their differences will be noticed by our society. It is their way of learning. It is their choice. We cannot all be on the same path. For them it is their chosen path and it is perfect for them. There is no right or wrong to life. There is only the IS of BEING. No matter what beliefs we attach ourselves to, what mind images we follow, they are all open for change if we are open and growing. Life is CHANGE. *The Universal secret to growth is true open-mindedness and the willingness to change.* Beliefs are necessary in our world. They are the fabric that molds our physical development. But beliefs need to always be viewed with open-mindedness. We must be willing to acknowledge when a belief has become an outgrown system for us and we must be open to changing that belief if we want to grow and change to the next level in our life. If we owned a car that was manufactured forty years ago and no longer runs, we would buy a new one. Sometimes it is essential that we buy a new attitude.

For those who become so attached to a belief that they refuse to turn loose of it, or refuse to even imagine perceiving it another way, the lesson of the belief may be the very lesson that they are here to work out in this lifetime. Many beliefs we humans live by are the beliefs of society and religion, which means that our beliefs are not unique to us. We are taught to do certain things, think certain ways, plan for certain events and to see our role in the world or our society in a certain manner. In most cases we are following ancient tradition that has been well worn and unchanged.

Our society spends billions of dollars reminding us to hold on to those beliefs. Many of us react to our religions, television, newspapers, radio, books, and other people like puppets on a string. We believe everything we are exposed to. This, too, is part of the belief system that we have learned. We will have learned a valuable lesson when we can choose our exposure and filter the information we must be exposed to, to only that which works best for us. It is each individual's singular choice to choose his individual belief system. We need to exercise our right of choice, our free will, in choosing exactly what works best for us. It is part of our human belief system that dictates that we must follow another person's beliefs.

Believing everything in our world breeds total confusion and sends mixed energy messages to the physical body. The five senses were given to us as our filtering system for the physical self. The most valuable tool to allow us to accomplish this filtering process in this physical life is the free use of the intuitive mind. If you sense the energy of the exposure as negative, filter it out of your consciousness. Protect your thinking mind from the physical reality of negative exposure. When we find our mind torn between an overload of conflicting and negative information, we become the energy of the negative conflict. We need to make a choice and see how it feels to choose. If choosing does not feel comfortable, it is easy to do as we have done in the past and attach ourselves to someone else's belief system, or to live our acceptance.

Choices, Alternate Paths, Probable Realities

No one is stuck in anything in life. The Universe has alternate paths for every situation. In Universal terms these are called probable realities. Your present reality is what you are doing right now. Your probable realities are the many other choices that are open for you, if you make a decision to take another path in life. The energy will always be there for you to use at will. Energy will be designed by you as an outlet if another energy channel becomes blocked.

We have free will. Approach what you do with love and you will get love in return. If this is not your reaction, then choose another reality. Your lessons are your lessons of choice. All of life will be whatever you perceive it to be and create it to be. These years of development set the approach that you will have toward your physical reality. They will be confusing years if they are approached with confusion. The mind is in the process of development so allow it to build with the positive energy of love. Let it be open to new ideas, new concepts and new people. Let the old stereotypes be what they may be and you be what you want to BE. If you can learn in this period of your life that it is okay to be different, the rest of your world will be full of light and happiness. You can let the JOY flow. You can freely accept the responsibility for who you are and who you want to be. You will change. Life is change, and if we refuse to change then we, in effect, die, although the physical death may take several years.

The goal of life is JOY and HAPPINESS in the Living.

During this time span these changes will bring about a total revision of your physical cellular structure, just as they have in every period of the Law of Sevens. Each of you is changing and those changes will be directed by the mind with the motivation of the Spirit. You have the ability to make your physical self what you want it to be. It requires the intent of the mind and the will to do what needs to be done, to make it a vital part of your reality. This is a period of too much drinking and too much eating of rich food. It is a period of not enough sleep. It is a period of drugs, alcohol and lust. It is a period of building the mind, and ignoring the body. It is a period of excessive work and play.

We need many things in the balancing act of life. We need work, play, love, caring, sharing, friends, beliefs, imagination, and Spirit. We cannot live on work alone without developing fear and depression. Love is an essential food for the body during all of life. Love needs to be given and it needs to be received. Love is not lust. Lust does not provide the caring and sharing, the communication, the knowing that someone thinks you are great just the way that you are. Love is food for the Soul.

One who feels love will have a better chance to eat right, sleep more appropriately, and to share and communicate. This provides a more stable grounding for development.

Nature's foods, for this period, are essential. This is a period of the drama of stress. Stress on the physical self activates stress within the cellular self. There is no escaping this action. The body is not capable of producing from any other foods one of the essential elements needed to fight stress in the human body. This element is Ascorbic Acid or Vitamin C. Vitamin C is found naturally in the fruits and vegetables grown in the sun's energy and should be consumed in large quantities. Nature's foods will provide you with all the essential elements including the germicidal properties that are crucial to you during this period of your development.

The stresses of our world are more than they have ever been on the physical self, because of the dramas we as a human species are creating. These dramas expose us to the elements that ravage the body. The body will struggle through some of the stresses, by making do and creating, but the cellular structure will suffer. Be consciously aware of what you eat and drink. Eat the fruits, vegetables, nuts, grains, and seeds of Nature and eat them in the closest form to Nature that is possible. Avoid large amounts of fat and sugar. Avoid processed foods, which contain additional fats, sugars, and chemicals. Nature's food will provide you with roughage to clean your body and the natural elements of Nature to restore and maintain your cellular function. Avoid drugs and excesses in alcohol. Make the time to sleep and to play. Think happy thoughts.

A mind that is directed only towards the material world will have tremendous conflict with the Spiritual self. He/she will feel the imbalance although he/she will not usually identify the true conflict. Pent-up feelings and emotions will manifest themselves in obsessive work and perhaps excessive play. Material possessions may become an obsession for the mind. The need for bigger and better toys will be the motivation he/she feels for work. Status and recognition will be the yearnings of the ego.

This period will be equally motivated by the opposite sex. The yearnings will continue for creation and pleasure on a physical level. For some this yearning will be motivated by a desire for constant approval. For some it will be the fear of being alone. For many it will culminate in togetherness. For many the fear of togetherness will produce aloneness. We will always look for approval in the belief system in which we are grounded. We may not recognize that JOY is not in our present belief system. The focus on status and belief systems in our society has led many Souls to choose other than their Spiritual mates as life partners.

A lack of awareness of self breeds confusion in the mind of all of humanity. It slows development of the Soul in the positive energy flow of awareness and understanding while lessons are being learned. That, too, must be for some Souls, primarily because some Souls need to slow down. We will continue in the space for both physical and mental attraction with the opposite sex. The degree will vary from person to person and from male to female. But for nearly all Souls, the mind will generate a stronger influence in their choice of mate now than at any other period of life.

Business becomes status and status becomes money, and money becomes status and business, and the circles of life continue. The material world is in full bloom. Even status is now an entity within itself in our world and can generate its own money and business. During this period it is possible to become a slave to work rather than working for the love of work. Material want changes the category from fun to work, to necessity. We do not live in a way that makes change easy for us. We begin to feel trapped by the reality that we have created for ourselves. This is "the stage of life" and we are reading, writing, and acting out our own human dramas.

Where is the peace? Where is the joy? Where does it all end? These are very personal questions that every person must ask. This drama of life does not usually end in this period of the Law of Sevens. We are so thoroughly engrossed in the drama of life that we, too frequently, miss the living. What we are doing, and how we are living, is to us the all-important issue. We are not worried about our body and our Soul because our ego is happy and truly enjoying an intriguing moment of power in time. Unfortunately, this period is frequently a time of self-aggrandizement, manipulation, greed, selfishness, and personal physical abuse. It is a time with a purely self-directed focus. It is a time for the ego to shine. It is a time of dramatic Spiritual Unawareness.

But always there is a light, somewhere in the darkness, that reflects the caring and loving Soul within. We cannot deny the integration of the body, mind and Spirit, even if we try, especially on a Soul level. When we attempt to erase the caring from our life, the need will become greater. This need will keep us focused on the imbalance until we will not be totally comfortable no matter how successful we become. The subconscious or Soul level of self will know that it needs to be recognized for the beauty of self internally and not the external trappings of status and money. The Soul memory will surface frequently enough to start the search once again in life.

During this period the search is usually conducted in the outer world, for the external, material wants of life. These material needs may be all that we are aware of at this period in our life. Our Soul sensing is there but the coordination of mind and Spirit has an incomplete bridge. Man will look for woman, woman will look for man. Man and woman may decide that it is their career that is not fulfilling. Some may decide that they need bigger and better toys. Few will recognize that it is within them that they must search for the answer because our Dual Soul and Spirit answers cannot be found externally. They are energy changes.

During this period of building and development, which is vital to the completion of this Soul journey, we are functioning primarily from the intellectual mind and the ego. The bridge to the body and Soul are not part of this present reality. The focus is singular and complete in our mind as we live and thrive in the material world. This is an illusion. There are no answers on the outside. All of the answers that are sought for a lifetime, by each and every Soul on Earth, are within the Soul consciousness and understanding of that individual core self in relationship to the physical.

As the fifth period draws to a close, in the first cycle of our life, awareness is there waiting to be acknowledged and invited in.

LAW OF SEVENS: **Sixth Period**

The sixth period of the Law of Sevens is the time between your thirty-sixth and forty-second years of life. This is a time of awakening and confusion. It is a time of continued development and the beginning of awareness. It is a time of continued searching. It is a time, in our Earth consciousness, of the beginning of mid-life crisis. Suddenly, the plans that you have formulated and developed during the past life period do not seem to be exactly right. You can't truly define what is not right but you have that "anxious" feeling. You have that "something is missing from my life" sensation. You have the need to search and understand yourself, more than you have ever felt it before.

This sense of imbalance is the Soul awareness that we create when we have developed either the physical, mental or Spiritual self out of synchronization with the other two trilocular units. After thirty-six years of focusing on the intellectual or the physical or the Spiritual, the self is confused and uneasy. It recognizes the imbalance and begins the search for the missing something. This search is the continuation of the search for balance that essentially begins at the moment of birth. We seldom recognize this search for what it truly is. But in searching for balance, we are searching to understand, to be aware of who we are and how we, as human beings, truly fit into the Universal Plan – the plan of an energy that is greater than us, the plan of Spirit.

We seldom define our uneasiness as a search for self or for Spirit. We continue our aggressive search for the physical and the material of life. We seek a new mate, a new job, a new location, a new exterior image, a new house, and a new car. This search can be endless as we focus our needs in the external world. This sixth period of life is the time when we look to our conquests. We search for more money, more fame, more sex, more women/men, more toys, and we begin our boundless search for what we believe to be our lost youth. There is that innate sense that IT was there, somewhere in the years past, and IF we can find "IT" we will at last be happy again. As both men and women grow through these same feelings, we are frequently living lessons that were uncompleted in our last lifetime.

This is a time of focusing on professional, family, and societal status. It is a time of knowing emptiness and loneliness. It is a time of searching. It is a time of abundance and need. It is a time of hard work and hard play. It is a time when we understand the world around us better than we understand ourselves. During our human life on Earth, we are primarily physical and we must function primarily from the physical reality. That is the Law of Nature, and the human being is a part of Nature. It is a Universal Law. We cannot be human if we deny the physical reality of life and living. We are a creation from the Earth. No matter what laws we create for ourselves we cannot erase the reality of our physical design and our relationship to Nature and Earth. We are and we will always be at our best when we are functioning within the rhythm of Nature and Earth.

When we attempt to remove ourselves from the laws of Nature, which functions with perfect balance, we will always be unbalanced. The human being is not a simple organism. We are a highly complex and constantly changing organism. Nothing can be said about us that will apply to all individuals always at a defined time. Nothing on Earth is absolute, because Earth is designed to change and grow. The words in this book are not absolute for all of eternity. There is a fluid connectedness to the energy of our Spiritual reality that constantly increases the positive and makes each living thing better than it was before. All increases constitute change, just as all decreases will constitute a dramatic change in the energy flow. As human beings, we are first and foremost "energy" beings.

The human is his own Dual Soul and Spirit Energy living in physical matter. Our Dual Soul evolution lives eternally within our own "sense" of being human. But the human being is an organism of Nature, in tune with Nature. When we acknowledge this relationship our attunement will change and evolve in a more completely balanced progression, expansion, and growth. Our human search will suddenly become a different search. It will develop an internal focus. We conduct our search based upon the degree of uneasiness that we are experiencing in our personal life. We design our search based on our belief system, knowledge, Soul memories, and our current level of mind awareness. If our belief system and our accumulated knowledge far overbalance our awareness level, we will design our search totally within the physical world that we know, and remain unaware that we live because of our energy.

We may frantically explore new ways to make money, searching for greater status. We may frantically explore the opposite sex, searching for the perfect partner that will make us feel complete on the inside. We may accumulate more and more possessions until we own millions of dollars and collectibles. We may read and study frantically, collecting and storing more and more information in our mind and in our physical collections. Whatever our search may be, if it is conducted from an unbalanced perspective of self, it will continue to produce an unbalanced result. The conscious physical self will remain unbalanced in relationship to the core self. This state of imbalance will motivate us to continue with our search, allowing it to take us wherever the search for life goes.

The True Reason for Our Need to Search

In this search that we find ourselves involved in during the sixth period of life, possessions will not count in creating a balance. Material possessions are of the physical. They are not of man. Possessions, whether they are material or professional, can be used as an effective method of avoidance in this search. This material search is a common human focus. We are noteworthy in our creation of physical need and physical activity for avoidance. The closer the thinking mind moves towards an awareness of the true development of the search for balance within the self, the more creative the ego becomes in protecting itself. During this period of life, we begin to create that internal tug of war that is the eternal struggle between the ego and the Dual Soul. This struggle is the true basis of the uneasiness that we can find in our physical reality. This ego, Soul conflict is the true reason for the need to search. It is the reason for building our mind and our body. This is the absolute lesson of life in our Soul evolution.

Everything that we have done thus far in our life, we have done to promote our own Soul evolution, our honest understanding of ourselves and how we truly fit into the overall picture of human life. Having reached this level of living without having true consciousness of our role in life makes us very uneasy. You are not alone in your search. Everyone who chooses incarnation on Earth is searching for his/her identity as an integrated part of his Dual Soul growth. Our true identity is the recognition of our Dual Soul. It is consciously discovering the Dual Soul memories to understand with conscious awareness all that you have been and will be as an evolving human being.

We are searching to learn the Spiritual balance of the physical body, Dual Soul mind and loving emotions, and the purity of our Spirit Self. If we were capable of learning this lesson in one day or one week, we would have no need to return to Earth countless lifetimes to continue with this eternal search. Learning the balance, the Dual Soul understanding of the love that Spirit is, and the love that we are striving to be, is a continuing lesson for all humans. When we understand that total unconditional love of "thyself as Spirit and thy neighbor as thyself," we will understand our mission on Earth. At that precise moment in our evolution, the Human will become pure of Spirit and will need no further Earth incarnations. By virtue of your choice to be human, you demonstrated your willingness to search for this understanding. For those who reject this mission, it is rejected on a conscious ego level, not a Dual Soul level. The resistance to being open to understanding ourselves is an intellectual or ego resistance that reinforces the struggle between the ego and the Dual Soul.

There are those who have intellectual reservations to loving "thyself as Spirit," because they do not feel worthy of comparing themselves to "Spirit" as they define Spirit. Their religious teachings have led them to believe that Spirit would punish them for entertaining such blasphemous thoughts. When we learn to love ourselves as Spirit, we are loving ourselves in the identical way and degree that we love Spirit. This love is and must be unconditional love. Loving ourselves unconditionally means that we do not judge ourselves, feel guilty, hate ourselves, or fear change. We know and acknowledge to ourselves that nothing we do, think or say is the reality of the total self except that elusive but overwhelming love within us.

In the everyday physical reality of our daily life, we will not be perfect. In the core self we are perfect. The struggle to perfect the mind is our struggle to learn how to perfect ourselves. It is the ability to BE Spirit-like in the mind that will build the bridge of understanding between the three units of self. When all humans learn to love our neighbor as ourselves, we learn to love ourselves unconditionally. Loving that which we do not possess or own, do not understand, or perhaps even know, is love that is given unconditionally. In our physical reality, we have an intense relationship to the energy of Spirit that we do not recognize because we are living our physical design. We have been taught by our belief system to love Spirit, even if we can't physically see "Spirit energy."

Unfortunately, Spirit has been dramatized by our religious society as a master that will punish us with hell and damnation, keep us from the gates of heaven and many other threats of anger. This is not an image of Spirit that Spirit has created. This is an image of Spirit that we have created. We have created an image of ourselves, in this image of Spirit that we have created, because we believe in sin and punishment. To Spirit we are a child and Spirit helps us, loves us, guides us, but does not punish us. We create our own punishment. We have a consistent habit of being hard on ourselves for what we view as our "transgressions" or "sins." When we believe that Spirit loves us and our Spirit's goal is to teach us to love ourselves in that same way, we begin to understand the truth of our own personal energy on a different level. This is the lesson of the heart. It is the lesson of love. This is the search for understanding self. Loving self is an awareness of us as perfect at the core of self as a Dual Soul and Spirit level of energy, despite the physical dramas that we have created. It is this awareness and love of thyself that allows us to act with love, to think with love and TO BE love.

Understanding yourself is loving yourself.

True understanding is not possible without that balance of love for which all humans are searching. We progress by levels in all things. When we truly love ourselves, we can truly love another person. The opposite is also true. If we do not love ourselves, we will be unable to completely, fully, and unconditionally love another person. But we can, as a physical person, know physical sex and physical lust. *These emotions are from the level of physical consciousness and are not the same sense of loving as a true love of the heart or Spirit Consciousness.*

It is during this period of life that man is intensely searching for that internal balance, that love of self. It is during this period that we also create many dramas for ourselves. We create dramas in proportion to the lessons that we need to learn. These life dramas become the life crisis in the world of someone who does not truly love himself. We create physical, psychological, mental and emotional dramas during this period that have become the basis of our sex scandals and entertainment world. We put the illusions of love on the screen which allows each of us to live them over and over again in our thinking mind on a daily basis. Whatever internal trauma we can't think of, someone will help us create.

We do much of our searching "for love" today very freely and openly as physical sex. We physically transmit the message of throwing away the old and searching for the new. This is the physical action that follows the mental concept. It is the physical action of the physical world. We throw out what we feel we are tired of living. In our world today, we do not acquire possessions or relationships that we intend to love and cherish. We acquire people and things in our life with the mental concept of discard, when they have served their usefulness to us for the moment. This mental concept of "throwing away" has a direct reaction on our physical body which is increasing our health problems.

Our Search for Something New

In our search for something new, we throw away relationships, physical possessions, professions, beliefs, and indeed our sacred human body. The mind is the builder. If the mind is in the concept of discard, as the perception of removing structures, it will also be removing the structures of the body, such as the thinking mind. Let us for a moment take from the Universe the reality of one person. We will deal only with a minute moment in this person's world. This is a professional man of considerable financial wealth. He has everything that he has ever wanted in his life. He graduated from all the right schools. He has the right "wife," not partner. He belongs to the right clubs. He is in the right profession. He has all the right toys but he is miserable. He doesn't feel as happy as he wants to feel. "Something" is missing. He isn't loved as much as he wants to be loved. There is no spark anymore. He needs something new. He needs a new wife, someone young, someone who will make him feel alive and free. Maybe a new car and a new house. Let's get rid of all of these old structures of life. He is ready to start over, to build a new life.

These thoughts that allow our man to start throwing away the old to build a new life, begin to throw away the physical self. These thoughts react within the body. The structure of the body is bone, blood, cells, and systems. Throwing away structure means depleting calcium and other minerals within the body. Depleting minerals means bones start to disintegrate, blood pressure begins to rise, and the heart begins to beat too fast, the blood changes, the cells change, other systems change. The body is throwing away the old. It is starting a new life. The mind has created dis-ease within the physical self. This is a demonstrated response of building the body with the mind. Our man may not have reached the point of acting upon his search for the new self on an external basis, but his thoughts have begun to create the change internally, which is compromising his health without his realizing the precise challenges that he is creating for himself.

When the physical body is subjected to any stress in the thinking mind, it must be protected by the balance of Nature's elements being provided internally. We must replace the ravages of stress with the proper food from Nature, to maintain the physical balance of our cellular design and structure. Maintaining the physical balance will allow us the freedom of health to balance our intellectual and Spiritual self. This search that we are unconsciously seeking in this sixth period of our physical life is an overall search for understanding ourselves and our place within our world. It is common at this point in our lives to seek the company of those who are younger than us because we see our age as a detriment rather than an asset.

As we mature, we will develop an awareness that our world is more than what we envisioned. We will understand that we are more than what we envisioned.

Near the end of this period, we will become restless and at conflict with the world that we see. We will feel at a loss to identify our feelings or ourselves. Our body will begin to suffer the effects of our conflict. Our searching is beginning to move from the unconscious to the conscious level of our intellect, and we are reaching out to new images of the physical to console ourselves.

In the third period of life, we see our capabilities and feel a sure sense of direction. In the sixth period of our life, our capabilities and our direction become clouded with internal conflict and confusion. We are not as certain that we are who we had envisioned ourselves to be. Maybe, just maybe, there is something that we don't understand about our world. Doubt in our chosen course begins to gnaw at our mind and heart. This is a truly creative period of life. It is a time of learning that there is more to explore both without and within. It is the necessary dark before the dawn of true creativity. It is the time when learning to love the self will allow us the freedom to grow and to BE. It is the first period of life, when there is truly a sense that there is more to life than simply the physical world that we create on a daily basis. It is a period that many live with total confusion and with minimal concern for loving thyself and thy neighbor. There are no lessons in life that are learned more clearly than those that are difficult.

When we design our physical world, we do it in such a way that we make ourselves work hard for what we learn. We set ourselves up to judge ourselves, even more harshly than others will judge us. Life is an unconscious judgment for us at this time. In reality there is no judgment, because Spirit does not judge. We create the illusion of judgment by our belief in right and wrong, good and bad. But as humans, made in the image of Spirit, we cannot do that which Spirit does not do. Spirit does not judge. We created the belief that we are being judged by Spirit. If we had not created a belief system for ourselves that designates everything into a category of either right or wrong, there would be no judgment. There is no right or wrong. There is only the IS of the NOW of your BEING.

Once the Ego and the Core Self begin the struggle for balance, there can be no turning back.

For all humans, the search is in the future of progress. The search has been unconsciously acknowledged and it will continue until we reach the end of this journey on Earth. In the next period of our existence, it will become even more of an issue in the reality of life. At last, there is a glimmer of an awakening. The awareness of the core self is starting. The search is now a reality for us and this conscious search will continue. Once the ego and the core self begin the struggle for balance, there can be no turning back. This sixth period of the Law of Sevens is the period of awakening for many. We are individuals, and no two humans are the same. No two people evolve in the same identical way at the same identical time. There cannot be a precise pattern of life that each person can define. But within the range of life, each person will find his own stages.

The sixth period is a period that may be experienced at any time in life, but for most it will be within its own range. The sixth period is a period of Soul growth for all of us. It is a time of opening to the consciousness of the Dual Soul. This growth experience depends upon an awareness of the Soul memory and an acceptance of the eternal evolution of the Soul. The Soul is always Dual as a thinking mind and loving emotions; therefore, we must evolve through the thinking mind into the loving emotions before we can understand ourselves and the world that we live within. In the midst of the confusion and the searching, there is a Soul memory that won't be denied. The Soul is down there, deep inside our unconscious mind. The challenge is to give that Soul the freedom to emerge. The sixth period is the true awakening of the Dual Soul of each human being.

LAW OF SEVENS: **Seventh Period**

The "Blooming" Stage of Being

The seventh period of the Law of Sevens is the period between the forty-third year and the end of the forty-ninth year. In the concept of growth it is the period of change. It is during this seventh period that man changes more of his concepts of the world and himself, than at any other period in his Earth life. It is the continuation of the awakening of his internal Dual Soul memories. The awakening of the Soul memories, that began in the sixth period, has now reached the "blooming" stage of being. Suddenly there is a need to be open to hearing the multiple concepts of Being. The search, that began with self, now intensifies and reaches out to the Universe for help in understanding.

This is the time for completion of the first cycle of the Law of Sevens. We have progressed from birth to fifty in this Cycle of Development. Our focus has progressed from the physical to the unity of the intellectual, to a developing awareness of the Spiritual. Now the time has come to complete the cycle, by balancing the body and mind with the Spirit. At last we are ready to look at the finite in terms of the infinite. The Spirit has stayed quiet and safe, in the knowledge of its own self. It has not been threatened during the time of development for the body and mind.

We are Spirit, as the eternal self. Earth incarnations require a physical body. The physical body can only be developed by the functional eternal mind. The Spirit has contributed the motivation of life, without being obtrusive with its presence. To do more at an early age, without the Soul memory of self, would create an imbalance that could not be handled by the physical self. This happens in our world and many of these Souls are considered mentally ill by those who have a belief that we live only one physical life. They are out of intellectual balance. Society, as it is today, does not know how to deal with this imbalance. Our "treatment" of chemical imbalance is primarily limited to drug therapy. Imbalances can be caused from any of the three trilocular units. Understanding this problem will change with the evolution of awareness in our minds.

These individual units of self are locked together at birth. Development of the three units, the mind, the emotions, and the sensory self, to their maximum level requires a lifetime of growth. As we develop the units begin to integrate, to slide closer into each other and lock more firmly into the position of total integration. We are three distinct circles of energy moving with a consistent centripetal force within each circle. But, each circle does not always move with the same degree of force as the other two. As the energy increases within each unit, the force increases until all units are moving with the same centripetal force. This uniform energy of each part integrates the parts of us into a tighter and tighter united energy force. This is the balance that we are seeking. We are now body-mind-Spirit. We are one being. We are whole.

The search for self began in the sixth period and will continue in this period as the Soul, as the core self, awakens. Our true self is our core self or Soul self. It is the Spirit self in each of us. It is that spark of energy, that seed of Spirit that we were created from and hold inherent within us that makes us human beings. It is this Spirit self within, that we came here to understand and to love. If we do not learn to love that Spirit within, that core self of our own being, we cannot learn to love Spirit. We cannot truly LOVE anyone else in our world, including ourself, until we are willing to acknowledge that we are the perfection of the Spirit energy within.

Without that understanding of who we are, and a total appreciation of who we are, we will never be able to love, to understand or to appreciate the energy of Spirit that is within all that energy has created as life-form. If we can compare ourselves to the Spirit Energy in relationship to children, we can more easily define the relationship that we have to Spirit. In the beginning, Spirit created us. In the beginning we created sons. The relationship is maintained throughout life, in both instances. Our son may deny our existence and choose never to speak to us again, but we are still his father. We may deny the existence of Spirit and never speak to Spirit again, but the Spirit is still the Creator of all that is human.

This is a true lesson of the heart. We must learn to love ourselves, before we can radiate that love, in the form of energy, to other people on Earth. Our lesson on Earth is to learn to love. Spirit is a loving energy, which helps us to understand that Spirit lives within each human being as love. To be in the perfection of Spirit we must learn how to live our love. It is the love of self, the awareness of us and Spirit, that creates the balance that we are seeking. It is loving thyself (physical), thy neighbor (mental), and thy Spirit (Spiritual) that balances the energy of the three units of self.

That message was given to us by Spirit, in the first two of the Ten Commandments. When we learn the lesson of love there will be no need for further commandments. The other commandments were written because of our lack of understanding of the first two commandments. It is our perception of Spirit that gave them their name. Spirit does not command. Spirit encourages and enlightens with love. The Spiritual message was: Learn to love yourself, me, and the rest of my creation. There is no one on Earth that we are closer to. Therefore, it is logical that the place we must start in learning love is within ourselves. We must look within to know who and what we are. We must look within to appreciate and validate our own core as the Spirit Self.

The entire realm of Earthly problems is the direct result of our not loving ourselves. The entire realm of individual problems is the direct result of our not loving ourselves. If we loved ourselves, we would love our neighbor, because we are one. There are no exceptions. If we truly love ourselves, then we can only radiate love to the world. We can only love our fellow man. The entire concept of reality functions from the trilocular concept of self. The concept of Spirit, as we now understand and accept, is the trilocular concept of Being. Spirit is "The Father, The Son, and The Holy Spirit."

"All men are created equal."

When we love ourselves we love the Spirit within and the Spirit within is our relationship to our fellow human. The Spirit within us is identical in all of us. "All men are created equal." This reference applies to the core self as the creation of the Spirit self. Our physical creation is our individual choice. When we love ourselves, we recognize our relationship to the living Earth that is our home. We see the Earth as the living matter that we are. We know the rhythm of the Earth as the rhythm of our physical body. We understand that the physical energy that we are comes from the energy of Earth, the mental energy that we are comes from the energy of Universal Knowledge, and the Spiritual energy that we are comes from the Spirit energy that is the energy of pure love.

Understanding the relationship of our physical body to the Earth will create miracles in this seventh period of Earth existence. The physical energy that has been stored by the body in the earlier years has been depleted. In our materialistic world, we have removed ourselves from the rhythm of Nature. We have spent years depleting the Earth elements that created the physical self and that allow it to function in a healthy, happy manner. The eventual result of body and mind imbalance is always disease. When we have created disease internally we cannot be free and joyful in living. Our physical and mental energy is out of balance. The action of this imbalance of body and mind creates the reaction of disease. Health requires a balance of energies. We are operating as physical energy beings in a physical reality. Therefore, it is crucial to our balance that the physical energy be maintained first and foremost to support our physical life, our health, and our happiness.

The physical energy of Earth is our core energy and it is our grounding energy. It is the energy that allows us to be human. Our physical energy comes from Mother Earth. The only way that we can take on and use this physical energy is to stay in rhythm with Nature. We need to spend more time restoring our physical energy by eating the natural plants of the Earth in their natural state, swimming in the waters of the Earth, breathing the pure air of the Earth. Digging in the Earth and growing plants of the Earth is essential to BEING. Being in physical relationship to the Earth is restoring Earth energy within our human body and it is always this Earth energy that creates and sustains the health of our human body, mind, and Spirit Self.

The mechanical, technical, materialistic society of Earth is breeding a society of humans that are quickly losing their Earth energy source. Loss of this Earth energy is loss of the physical, which has the ability to destroy the physical aspect of the human design. This is evident in our culture by the increase in disease and dis-ease. It is evident by the early onset of "old age" and the early deaths that are prevalent through disease. We create our diseases by the excesses and deficiencies of our Earth relationships (food, air, water) and our mental attitude towards living a physical life on Earth. With our creation of disease, we accept a further insult to our physical self by adding countless chemicals in the form of medicine, which we believe will cure our abuse. Any compromise to an already depleted physical self creates a more depleted self.

The energy source of the physical self is essential to physical life. For the self that has reached the seventh period of the first cycle of existence it is important to restore that physical self. We have the capability of truly advanced life on Earth, from the sense of Earth time and quality, if we choose to accept the responsibility for this capability. Advanced life on Earth cannot be "given" to us. It must be our heart's true desire to maintain the

"Earth energy" chemical structure within our physical self which is essential to support procreation.

The lesson of physical balance is an Earth lesson for all humans. It is a lesson that requires countless incarnations on Earth before the awareness is there to understand the need for physical balance. The lesson of integration is another of Earth's lessons. The lesson of integration is only possible after we have learned the lesson of physical balance. We are working our way up the ladder of evolution. The cycle of development consists of countless lessons of the physical self (body). This physical imbalance cannot be recognized by the physical form that we see, except through our definition of disease. Those with the capability of sensing will be conscious of extreme energy depletion and blockage before the onset of physical symptoms. This blockage can be felt and seen in the energy and physical body before disease can be defined by science.

Physical balance is seen in the conscious coordination of body and mind. It is seen in the ability to heal the body with the mind. It is seen in the energy field surrounding the body and the glandular energy that flows through the body. It is seen in the vitality of living and the peace of being. Integration of the body, mind and Spirit, as the three primary energy sources that we are designed to use, can free us of disease and emotional turmoil. For us to bloom during this seventh period of the first cycle of life, we must be open to the changes required for this integration to become part of our world. We have the capability of creating balance during this period more than at any other time thus far in our Earth life.

We have acquired the physical, the mental and now the Spiritual memory of existence. They are now part of our being and they are a part of our physical design. All that is left for us to do is to perceive them with the LOVE of self that is required for final integration. They must be recognized, used, and acknowledged. If we cannot do this, we are continuing to live in denial and resistance. We are proving to ourselves and the Universe that we are not humble enough to accept change.

Self-perception is looking within and loving. Self-perception frees us from the burden of time and space. It allows us to understand that we are eternal. It shows us that we cannot die. We are our core self, as the eternal energy of our Spirit. Self-perception is accepting that physical birth is the confining state that we have chosen to grow in and to learn in. It is realizing that we take on the clothing of the human body to be students in the Earth school. It is knowing that we have created the illusion of death as a means of controlling the actions of life. There is no death. Leaving the physical body is the choice that our human energy makes to regain and to restore our Spirit energy as our freedom. When we perceive a loss of freedom on Earth, death can be our choice of change. Birth is a confinement or partial death to the Spirit and it means giving up the mantel of the Spirit energy for the physical self, which allows us to see death as the return of total freedom to the Spirit self. Rebirth establishes our physical control.

Being open to the true perception of self and our relationship to the Universe in this period will entitle us to the peace and joy that every person is seeking, for our second cycle of existence. We can seek the balance of integration in a very structured and logical fashion in our world. We have learned discipline and structure. We are comfortable working within that discipline and structure. Realizing that we control this process and can approach life and death in an organized manner will help the Spirit motivate us to success.

Look At Your World

Look at your world. What is the physical condition of the self? How do you care for that self? Do you expose your body to the elements of the Earth to restore your energy? Do you rely upon modern medicine to keep your physical self alive? Do you balance your physical self with the foods of Nature in their natural state? Do you take the time from your daily activities to rest and to play? Do you work long hours and find your body tired and absent of true energy? Do you spend time with people, caring about them and sharing yourself with them? Do you give and receive love freely? Do you cherish your friends and know them as you know yourself? Do you appreciate the life that you have and the love that you have? Do you love yourself? Do you find JOY in your life? Do you laugh often and in total happiness at being alive and well? Do you sleep peacefully and awaken bursting with joy and love for yourself and the world? Do you feel that your internal energy is stable and supporting you in your life?

These are some explorations for looking within. When we look within we are viewing the integrated self, the core self, the intellectual self and the physical self. They cannot be separated. The integrated self always appears as one you. The self does not have to be totally balanced to be integrated, because the integration is there from birth. The balance is what we seek in the physical life that we are living. We are body, mind, and Spirit. We are three distinct and separate functioning energy forces. As we have been made aware in the different periods of life, we are focusing on the development of these different energy fields. Once they are developed we can begin the process of seeking our internal balance.

Our Creation of Self and Our Earth Reality

Nothing in life is ever singular as we are born in a state of integration. Therefore the development, awareness and understanding levels are fluid, and flow at different rates in each of us. The balance, too, is different in each of us and that, too, is fluid within as it is without in our Universe. The understanding, awareness and openness to the living, to the balancing, to the searching, are the Soul motivation for learning about the self. The energy of the self flows through the physical, around the physical and within the cellular formation of the physical. This is our creation of self and our Earth reality.

Seeing our world from the physical, the intellectual and the Spiritual level will help us design our own questions. As the questions are reviewed internally, we will find areas of our life that we are content with and that we recognize as our grounding energy. These energy forces will be the good parts of our life that give us the will and intent to look within the deeper areas of our body, mind and Spirit. The good parts of our life are to be cherished. They should be validated by acknowledgement, valued highly, respected, appreciated and protected gently but powerfully with total love. They are our Earthly salvation. Do not allow them to disappear from your world. Nurture them tenderly and lovingly. They are the reinforcement of our own strength that will allow and encourage us to grow. They are love.

Looking within at the things we have chosen to forget will be the uncomfortable part of our searching. There is no other way to know the true self. The person you are is the person that you have made specific choices to become. If you find within things that are not comfortable, you have the choice of changing self. In this process of review, remember that you do it with total discernment. Do not judge yourself, or others. The past experiences of our life are exactly that, they are experiences. They were, and they are, opportunities for learning. The experience can be changed at any time that we choose to change it. There is no past. There is no right or wrong to the choices that we make. There is only the lesson that we need to learn from the experience. Our review is to understand the lesson of the experience. Without a complete understanding of the lesson, we will consistently repeat the experience.

During this seventh period of the Law of Sevens, we are searching for understanding and growth. We cannot grow if we are captured within a repetitious cycle of negative experience. Looking at the experiences and finding the thread of continuity that runs from one experience to the next will help define exactly what we are trying to learn. All lessons will be based in Universal Law. All lessons will filter down to the primary focus of our incarnating on Earth. This is the lesson of Love thyself, Spirit, and all that Spirit has created. Therefore, it is easy to define why we are here. We are here to learn to love. We are on Earth to learn to function and to live with the love of our Eternal Spirit in the physical plane. We are here to learn the balance that is created by love.

We do not see clearly in our experiences because we have learned to place blame. We have not learned that we are responsible for self. There is no one to blame. We have not learned to look within, to find the intent of self, because it may not be a comfortable intent. It may not be an intent that is based on love and service to humankind.

It may be a totally self-directed, self-focused, ego-controlled intent that will serve only our ego needs. When the intent is poorly focused, the blame will be placed on another who has agreed to share the experience. It will not be looked at from within, to find the true problem that the self has created for the lesson of the experience. In reviewing experiences, do not look to the other Souls involved in the experience with you. Their lessons are different from yours. It is of no concern in your own growth, to consider their experience. Look at why you chose this experience. What were you trying to gain in your own Soul evolution?

Soul evolution is never focused on material gain. The focus is only on the growth of the entire Dual Soul. Abundance is a secondary experience that will serve as another lesson in Soul evolution. Material gain is a physical reaction. Without the growth of the Soul there cannot be true abundance. True abundance has nothing to do with material possessions. Material possessions are temporary physical things. In the order of Soul evolution, abundance relates to that which can be retained within our Eternal Soul and Spirit. We can retain love within our Dual Soul and Spirit, but we will not be able to take our material possessions with us.

Each lesson must be learned in the order of the Universe. Many will read these words and immediately cite examples of people that are far from Spiritual but may enjoy tremendous abundance on Earth. We must not judge others or Spirit. When the lesson is complete in abundance, service becomes another lesson. The very lesson of physical abundance is a difficult lesson and may take many incarnations to learn. The accumulation of material possessions makes it more difficult to develop awareness and understanding because the ego is in control. Souls that are born into great wealth may be working on the lesson of abundance in this lifetime. Many who do not have abundance today may have completed that lesson during previous lifetimes.

Abundance is found in the many mansions of Spirit. On Earth, abundance is identified with material possessions. For those who have progressed through the lessons of the physical, material abundance may be viewed as a burden in this lifetime. If physical abundance is part of your life design of this incarnation, it will be provided. But you must complete the lessons that come before the one of abundance. If you do not progress as planned, the design of your lesson will be aborted and you will leave the physical plane with Karma for your next sojourn on Earth.

We should never fail to be aware of the abundance that is found in the Mansions of Spirit that have nothing to do with material possessions. Abundance is found in health, in friends, in family, in love, in physical balance, in caring, in sharing, in honesty, in guidance, in faithfulness, in openness, in truth, in relationships, in knowledge, and all the other mansions within that make us truly a child of Spirit. Reviewing the experiences of our life is an opportunity for Dual Soul growth. Despite the uncomfortable sense that we may experience with this effort, the lesson of searching within is important. This can be done with the knowledge of love of self that will help transcend the fear of separation that the mind feels in the process.

Looking within is best when done in quiet meditation. The energy of the Spirit will allow you to view these experiences of life in the brilliant light of understanding, which will provide insight for the conscious mind. The Spirit knows no time. Everything that has been, or will be, is available to us, within the light of the Spirit. The healing energy of this light will allow you to capture the true core self of your being, and understand with a conscious awareness the path of your Dual Soul. This becomes a cleansing of the mind and Dual Soul. It is the bridge that is formed to help you with your search for understanding and love. It is an opening up of the Universe that gives validity to your being in the physical.

Viewing physical reality in the light of Spiritual reality gives us a totally new concept of being. We begin to truly value self as a unique and vital energy source. We begin to understand the power of being. We begin to understand love. We begin to appreciate the Earth for the energy source it is for our physical self. We begin to understand the purpose of creation. We begin to feel a whole being. We begin to feel balanced. We begin to become conscious that we are more than just a physical body.

At this time in your life you are nearing the completion of the Cycle of Development. It has taken you fifty years of immediate experience to gain new insight into the self. This new awareness will guide you in your Soul evolution during the next cycle of life, which is the Cycle of Awareness. Our society defines the next fifty years of life as one of "old age" or senility. Spiritual understanding challenges that definition of being. If we truly understood how old we really are, we would be forever laughing at the young who refer to age fifty as old. It is only with the experience of age that we truly learn who we are and what we are growing into being. Age is an asset, not a detriment. We make age a detriment, by virtue of our belief system. The value of age has been totally lost in our society because of our belief system. This is a critical loss to our society of today. It is not something to be cherished, but it is something to be changed. The *down streaking* of the energy forces of the physical body is being created by the excesses and deficiencies of our society. Balancing our human lifestyle will allow our experiences to create rather than disintegrate.

The close of the Cycle of Development will find aware Souls excited to be entering a new cycle of their life. It can be the most creative and productive period of life for you when you know the value of love. With the closing of the Cycle of Development we enter a new cycle that is known in Universal terms as the Cycle of Awareness. If we have developed insight into the awareness that each of us has, then we will find this cycle the most enlightening and exciting cycle that we have reached in this incarnation. If we have failed to develop insight into the awareness of our Dual Soul, do not despair. It is never too late to open the mind of the Dual Soul to the Universal teachings.

This cycle will require that we look at ourselves as we have never looked before. It will require peace and tranquility. It will require joy and happiness. It will require love. Know the peace that you are entering. This is the school for the Dual Soul and Spirit of us as human beings.

SECOND CYCLE OF THE LAW OF SEVENS

The second cycle of the Law of Sevens is the beginning of the second season in our life on Earth. During the first fifty years of life, we are experiencing the Cycle of Development. During the second fifty years of life, we are experiencing the Cycle of Awareness. *All that we are is there at birth, but it must be developed in the Law of Physical Matter. We must learn to be human.* We have entered the realm of Earth, the realm of physical matter as a Spirit Consciousness. We cannot begin to approach the purpose of this lifetime, until we have developed in the ways of the physical. The energy that we are as Spirit has made the decision to assume human form for the purpose of our Dual Soul evolution. To assume human form this Spirit Consciousness must clothe itself in physical matter. The Spirit repeatedly designs a physical body for itself in the same way that we design clothes for ourselves as people.

No two designs will be totally alike. The cellular patterning is known to the Spirit. It is the pattern of energy that was designed by Spirit. The material design concept for the body is created by the core of self, the Dual Soul and Spirit Consciousness, to fulfill the purpose of the physical incarnation on Earth. Each incarnation for the Soul will require a human design that will allow that Soul to work through the purpose it has planned for this Earth existence. As the Soul enters the second cycle of being, the physical development has been completed. The mind and the Spirit have also developed, as they must, since we are integrated at the moment of birth. But this development has a lopsided appearance in the energy essence of being human.

Imagine Three Equal Circles

Imagine a super jet coming in for a landing. One tire on the plane is flat. When this plane touches the ground the energy force of the tires will be uneven. The unbalanced force will be so pronounced that the plane may crash. That is how we feel as we enter the second cycle of life. Imagine three equal circles. These circles are representative of the physical body, thinking mind/loving emotions, and Spirit Senses. During the cycle of development, one circle of energy may grow larger than the other two. Think of yourself and mentally create each circle the size that you find equivalent to the development that you acknowledge in each area of your body, mind and Spirit Consciousness.

These circles of energy overlap. The degree of overlap is equivalent to the degree of integration. Envision your own circles and the degree of overlap. This vision is where you are today, despite the physical age that you have reached. The second cycle of life is the Cycle of Awareness. We have gained the development that is necessary. We no longer need to focus on the physical development of self. The physical product is complete in structural design and form. Now we need to stand back and allow the Soul to observe the art of creation. Is it the best that it can be? The quality of self cannot be appreciated fully, until we are aware of the energy balance of self.

Within the Cycle of Awareness is a new search. What are we inside? Who are we inside? Are we only flesh, blood and bones? Are we only the career that we have created? Are we only the material possessions that have our life bulging at the seams? What is life all about? What does it mean to be alive? Is this all there is? Each and every second of life contributes to the growth of self in an integrated way. No growth can occur without affecting the total. As we enter life as a Spirit Consciousness, we carry within our Universal pattern the motivation of life, the Soul memories, the Universal knowledge, the awareness of purpose, and the love of Spirit and self.

During the conversion of the Spirit Consciousness to live in human form these memories are overgrown with the physical activity of our life. The overgrowth of the Dual Soul happens in the same way that a field will become a jungle of trees, bushes, and plants if it is left without loving care. As we live and are absorbed with the activity of life, our memories of the Spirit world become smothered with the "things" of Earth. Our focus becomes work, study, music, television, sports and other physical interests. There are also the frequent physical "love" interests that become an art and a sport for us as human beings. We forget to devote loving care to the Spiritual memories that lie dormant within our core self. Our thinking mind has become a jungle of thought and concern for the physical space that we know and love. The Dual Soul and Spirit Consciousness are living now as a physical human being. The activities and beliefs of life have taken priority for that life. It is a busy time! As physical development progresses, the mind is also developing and adding more material to cover the memory of the Dual Soul. As the belief system is established, the ego is flourishing and reaching its peak of being.

The information of our society feeds our ego to focus on the material, physical world. This is equal to spraying growth hormone on the foliage. The ground cover of the Dual Soul and Spirit Consciousness thickens and smothers the Soul memories further into the core self. The ego is in control, and the ego sees the Dual Soul as being in direct competition to its position of power. As we develop and move forward in our growing need to understand ourselves, we begin to search through that ground cover looking for the memories. Why do we suddenly begin that search? We begin searching because the state of imbalance that we have reached makes us aware of a missing piece that will keep the self balanced. Finding that balance suddenly becomes survival in the physical reality that we know. Even without a conscious concept of the energy forces that create the total self, we are still acutely aware of that sense of imbalance. We become a super jet operating with only two fully inflated tires. We feel the loss of power. We feel the danger that we have created. Our path is not smooth and we are searching. As the search progresses we develop an acute awareness of that functioning Dual Soul, that memory of self that is hidden under all the tangle of physical possessions, physical activities, and intellectual beliefs. In our need for that balance, we forge ahead in our search until we begin to break through the physical and the mental and we attempt to see the self as more than we had imagined. As we search we find it easier than we thought it might be. We may not understand in the beginning that we have the advantage of the Spirit Consciousness there to guide us in this all-important search for growth. But as we search, we feel new energies opening up and becoming part of our immediate physical world.

The Dual Soul is designing a program to Clean House

The core self is the internal pattern of our Spirit Consciousness that knows the time has come on all planes, to balance out this physical body that acts as the temple that it uses as a house on Earth. The Dual Soul is designing a program for cleaning house. The Soul is determined to break through the physical and intellectual ground cover. The Soul is ready to be recognized as an integrated part of the whole self. *This is the beginning of life that we create as a body, mind, and Spirit to help us learn the fine art of growth and change.*

Soul memory, for many human Souls, does not exist on a conscious level during this period of intense physical and intellectual involvement. But we can experience the effect of Soul memory on a physical level. This is the Spirit's way of maintaining an energy connection to that Soul memory in an Earth-focused Dual Soul. An example of this effect is the response that we have to the sun and the moon. When the sun is shining in all of its brilliance, our Soul is happier, more joyful and productive than at any other moment in life. Have you ever heard someone say, "When the sun goes down, I can't work anymore," or "I am a day person, I don't have any energy at night"?

The Soul memory relates to the brilliant light of the sun, to the brilliant light of the Spirit. Within the sun we find our lost Spirit, and we know peace. We find our motivation for living, we find true joy and we are at one within ourselves. The sun offers us that moment of balance that we are unconsciously searching for. When the sun is removed from us, for days or weeks or months, our minds will become fragmented, feel totally disconnected from the physical reality, be depressed, sad, angry and even suicidal. The connecting energy, the motivation of the Spirit that is the sun, has been removed. We have lost that thread of balance that the sun provides with the memory of our lost Spirit-Soul.

Our Earth has many sun worshipers. We will stay in the sun to the detriment of our own physical body, because we find peace when we are in the energy of that unconscious memory stream. In Soul memory, this sun worship is directed toward Spirit. Consciously, we have no awareness of the Spiritual relationship that we feel for the sun. The opposite is also true, with the Soul memory and the moon. A full moon images the separation of the Soul from the light of the Spirit. The Soul memory is of the body leaving the light of the Spirit, destined for Earth. The Soul is seeing that light grow dimmer in the distance. It no longer has the brilliance of the sun but as it fades into the distance it is an illumination. The Soul is conscious of no longer having the awareness of the brilliant energy streams, and no longer feeling the safety of this supporting energy.

The Root Cause of All Fear within Us

This is the first experience of fear that the Dual Soul encounters. The Soul memory of the moon then is the memory of the separation from "Spirit," which triggers the absolute fear of eternal separation from Spirit in our mind. This memory of the Spirit separating from us is the true basis of our fear of separation. This fear of separation from Spirit is the root cause of all fear within us. Our Soul immediately forgets that Spirit is not totally separated from us. We are overcome with loneliness and fear. We are overwhelmed by our role as a human on Earth. Remembering the eternal Soul is a lesson that we have come to Earth to learn.

We will respond to the moon by becoming overwhelmed with fear, and many times losing total control of our reality. Unconsciously, we are again suffering from the separation of Spirit Consciousness. Unconsciously, we are trying to remember that the Spirit continues to dwell within us. Unconsciously, we are trying to remember that there is nothing to fear, there is no separation. Unconsciously, we are trying to acknowledge the subconscious Soul self that lives within. We will experience this separation in varying degrees of unrest. We may be sad, depressed, suicidal, angry, and violent or any number of other negative emotions may surface on the conscious level. It is also at this moment that the body of the mother who is pregnant will decide to separate the two Spirits.

As the awareness level of the Soul increases, the dramatic effect of the sun and the moon on our physical self will decrease. Our enjoyment of both will increase in a direct relationship to our subconscious understanding of our role in the Total Universal Plan. An advanced Soul will find peace in the presence of the sun and moon, because we will view them as a true energy connection to our core self as Spirit Consciousness. At about fifty years of age, we leave the Cycle of Development and enter the Cycle of Awareness. The actual physical age is unimportant. Chronology of time is being used only to allow us to perceive the relationship of experience to our internal Dual Soul growth. We must be aware and open to understanding ourselves, before we can learn and experience progress in Soul evolution.

The lessons that have been understood are the growth experiences that allow us to progress into the second cycle of life. Many Souls will not enter the Cycle of Awareness, but will remain frozen in the Cycle of Development until they abort their life plan. For them this is not wrong. They are where they have grown to be. It is the perfect position for them. Soul growth is an internal process that cannot be suddenly created by that Soul on demand from any outside source. The internal need of the Dual Soul must initiate the growth. This does not mean that a Soul cannot accept guidance, if the need is recognized within the true self. When a Soul is ready for growth, it must only ask and the teacher will be there.

Physical age has nothing to do with the true growth of awareness. Some advanced Souls will enter Earth life with awareness. Others will develop awareness rapidly as they experience their physical lives, because it is a strong Soul memory. But for the sake of our explanation we will use the chronological cycle of life. There are many Soul cultures and Soul group cultures in the Spiritual world. Soul cultures are formed primarily by highly evolved Souls with the same or an interrelated Soul purpose. Soul cultures are mainly service cultures. They are teaching and healing cultures that spend numerous lifetimes incarnating together and working together for the service of the Universe, humanity and Spirit on Earth.

Group cultures are formed by younger Souls that may not at this point totally understand their Soul purpose. They need the comfort of group leadership and group activity. They will incarnate together many, many times in their efforts to learn and progress in Soul evolution. In the physical realm these Souls can be identified by their need to follow, to be in groups, to work for a cause. Souls from these cultures will attach themselves to gurus, ideas, and beliefs. They are not comfortable searching for their own reality of being. They do not, at this point in their growth, have the strength to be different. Souls from the group cultures will be extremely active in the realities of physical life. They are comfortable in an already defined reality. They gravitate to the realities created by society. Soul cultures will concentrate on thinking and group cultures will concentrate on doing. This cannot be accepted as absolute, because each and every Soul has the free will to spend his time as he designs. A Soul may choose to spend time with a group culture that is working on an interest that he can help with. Crossover is necessary for growth and is welcomed as an opportunity in the Spiritual world, to teach.

Soul cultures differ in respect to growth. The growth of one culture, now on Earth, is more advanced in Soul evolution than most cultures are. Soul cultures understand and want to be involved in certain realities that we have created. Souls form groups that incarnate together for a culture or group purpose, as well as their individual Soul purpose. These highly evolved Soul cultures incarnate together, when there is danger of destruction to the Earth or some mass lesson of the Spirit to be taught such as healing. The present advanced Soul culture on Earth has returned to be involved with both lessons at once. This decision was made, as a group purpose, for the Soul culture to heal the fear and teach the healing of love, which will allow the survival of Earth. Earth is constantly populated with many groups of Soul cultures. Today the culture that is on Earth to teach love is a very large and advanced culture. Many Souls in this culture are freely in communication with the Spirit/Souls on other levels. Many Souls in this culture can span the consciousness levels and help Earth in ways that are yet to be explained to most people, because their knowledge comes from their memory of past lives and their relationship to the land of Earth and its hidden capabilities in maintaining health within the human being. We have contaminated Earth to the point that Earth is harboring diseases.

Earth is a School, a Learning Center with many Classrooms

There are guides, Spirits, and incarnated Souls that are working daily to teach purification and cleansing of the Earth. Cleaning and purifying the Earth is working with the energy streams that hold the physical substance of the Earth together. Positive energy forms a cohesive bonding of all Earth substances. This energy flows in a smooth stream maintaining the balance of Earth. Negative energy will allow the substance of Earth to break down and fall apart. The uneven constricted energy stream can then block and squeeze the life out of Earth. Earth is a school, a learning center with many classrooms that were designed by Spirit for us as Spirit creations. Souls of these Spirit creations populate the Earth as we are working through various levels of our Dual Soul growth. We have our own separate realities, in our individual level of awareness. The Souls with highly developed awareness levels can and do interact with Souls on other awareness levels.

Some Souls that are now entering their Cycle of Awareness are preparing to teach love and healing. This teaching has already begun for many Souls, and is in progress in our world today. We will see an escalation of Spiritual teaching and awareness. Do not be afraid to listen. Each Soul has free choice of acceptance and denial. If the Soul has progressed enough in its growth, it will remember and understand the ancient Philosophical teachings. To increase this progress of Soul awareness and memory we must look within at our Soul growth and the understanding that we have gained from the experiences of life.

The beginning of the second cycle is the period of opening to Spiritual awareness for many Souls. It is a period of continued search for that identity, that balance within self. It is a period when awareness will set us apart, if we allow it to make us feel different. We are not different, we are growing. Resistance and denial of change is equivalent to chaining our physical body to a stone wall. These beliefs, chains, wrap around us, binding our arms, legs, head and torso securely to the stone wall. We cannot escape. If we choose to chain ourselves to our current belief system, understand that it is our choice to be chained to the stone wall of ignorance.

For those entering this period with a wondering of how to progress, that is easy. Understand that life is change. Be open to change. Be open to learning. Be open to growing. Do not cling to preconceived ideas about anything. Open your mind, your heart and your Spirit. Let it soar. Let it be free. Let it feel. Trust in the Universe. Leave the decisions to the Universe. Turn loose of the ego control of your life. Allow yourself to grow and change as the personification of your internal Spirit Consciousness Energy.

The first change that we must make to develop awareness is to learn about self. We cannot learn about self in the daily noise and activity of life. We must be willing to remove as much negative input from our world as we possibly can, without taking ourselves totally away from our physical reality. Spend time when you have no radio on, no television, no one talking to you. Find alone time in Nature whenever it is possible. Look within, know yourself. Think about who you are and what you want, from the level of the Soul rather than the level of the material. Meditate. Meditation is an internal Soul communication. It is a communication of the physical you and the intellectual you with the Spiritual you. It can be done anywhere and at any time. If you need structure to facilitate the process, develop a structure.

As you progress in your level of awareness, you will find yourself in communication with your Dual Soul and with other Souls. You will begin to function from the heart-mind link. The male is seeking to link to the body of self. The females need additional grounding. The males are grounded but have a difficult time feeling and sensing from the Spirit self, because of their attachment to the physical. The results of this linkage are apparent and constantly operating. Men marry for primarily physical attraction; women marry for love as an emotion. Women want to get married because they are seeking grounding. Men don't want to get married because they are seeking physical gratification through sex.

We often say that there is a difference between the male and female mind. This is not accurate. The Universal knowledge is available to all. The difference between man and woman is the perception that is created by the mind-heart linkage. Women assimilate thought through the heart or Spirit self. Men assimilate thought through the supreme physical sense of self. This mind-body linkage, and mind-Spirit linkage is very pronounced in the early years of life. As the Soul matures, the priorities of the person change with the new balance that is created. If both male and female are of equal growth in terms of Soul balance, a relationship has a better chance of survival within our physical world.

Choose Wisely

Having a partner that is willing to grow with you is a perfect way to strengthen relationships. Spend quiet time together. Practice positive communication on a Soul level. Understand each other. Quiet down your lifestyle. Limit your reading to positive information. If it makes you laugh, enjoy it. If it relates nothing but war on any level, turn it aside and search for the positive reading of understanding and growth. Know that you have a choice of what your life truly is. Whatever you do, whatever you say, however you feel, however you think are all your individual choices. No one makes your individual choices for you. Every human has free will. Choose wisely.

It is with the loud music, the constant talking, the constant doing, and the constant searching for news of the world and others, that we allow ourselves to lose sight of us. We understand the political world better than we understand the world of self. How can we make decisions that affect the Universe, when we can't make decisions about what we should do in the next moment, what we should wear, what we should eat for dinner, or which television program we want to watch? This is why we need to mix the males and females together in important aspects of decision-making. Balance works well when it is used in thinking and doing to create our world and enjoy our lives.

The process of understanding and awareness is an internal process. It cannot be conducted as a scientific research project that studies other people. We must first study ourselves internally, from the physical matter that we created as body, to the functioning mind, to the core self of our Soul and Spirit. Our Soul and Spirit are the eternal energy that allows us to live many human lives. We are designed to look within for the answers which will always be found in the accumulative energy of our core self that we have created through our many lives as we have lived on Earth.

True emotional health is Spiritual growth. It is allowing those Soul memories to surface. It is understanding that we are more than our physical manifestations. It is being aware of why we are here on Earth. It is accepting responsibility for the creation that we are. It is loving, sharing, caring. It is oneness. It is honesty, truth, faithfulness, open-mindedness, trust. It is non-judgment in a world of opposites. It is loving yourself. It is finding your balance of trilocular energies. The beginning of the second cycle of life is the time for YOU. It is the time for ACCEPTING YOU. It is the time for BEING. It is a time for listening to the inner you, the Soul that wants to be heard. It is the time to balance YOU and to live your true emotional health.

In the Book of Spirit, Spirit tells his creations, "There is a time for all seasons…" This was a reference to the cycles that exist for all and everything within the Spirit

Kingdom. Earth is the Kingdom of Spirit. We are major actors in that Kingdom. There are four seasons of Earth, and there are four seasons of our human life. As we enter the second cycle of life we are entering the second season of our existence on Earth. There are four seasons of Nature and there are four seasons of man. On today's Earth, we fail to maintain the balance of energies required to enjoy the complete cycle of all four seasons. But we have the capability, with growth through awareness and understanding, to experience four seasons of Earth life during some of our physical lives.

The Law of Compensation, Balance

In the Cycle of Awareness, we will be experiencing the Law of Compensation. "There is a time to sow, and there is a time to reap..." and if the seeds we have sown are seeds of love, we will reap love. If the seeds that we have sown are seeds of hate, we will reap hate. If the seeds we have sown are seeds of self-abuse, we will reap disease. What we give we will eventually have returned to us, in another season of life. All energy flows in circles. Eating is the main cause for our reaping disease, because the design of eating from Nature has been lost through our scientific growth as a human species. The Law of Compensation is a Law of Balance. If the balance does not occur in this sojourn, it will have to be dealt with in another lifetime. That is the "Karma of life," fulfilling the Law of Compensation. "There is a time to sow, and there is a time to reap." As we have lost the knowledge of eating from the soil, we have interfered with our internal chemical balance. Awareness allows us to live a life that will not produce Karma or negative compensation. Awareness allows us to work out our life design, and clean the slate for the next incarnation. Awareness allows creation, through increased understanding and knowledge, in how to live a healthy life.

The Karma of life is not an act of Spirit. It is a human act. Spirit does not tell us what to do. We have free will. In that identical concept we are not protected from the mistakes we choose to make. Spirit allows us to learn by our own choice, at our own speed. Our life, now and forever, is solely of our own physical creation. We cannot credit the influences of mother, father, spouse, lover, children or anyone else, for the person that we are and the actions that we take. *We are who we have designed ourselves to be and our understanding of life becomes apparent to us and to other people in the way that we live our life.*

Reaching the level of awareness allows us to accept the responsibility for the creation of self. Accepting the total responsibility for the creation of self gives us the freedom of change. If we continue to blame another person for the person that we are, we fear change, because change will require that we accept personal responsibility for ourselves. If we accept personal responsibility, we will not have the safety net of blaming someone else. Placing blame is a fear of accepting responsibility. Placing blame is merely a symptom of the deep-rooted fear of separation that is overwhelming in our society. With the freedom of change we can look within the true self, and make the changes that will give us the peace of awareness. We can remove the stresses of our emotional and physical life, by changing the perception we have of the people and events which we encounter every day. The perception we have of any and all situations in our life creates the reality of the physical situations in our life.

Our Perception Creates Our Reality

An example of this creation by perception is the relationship that you have with the people with whom you spend eight hours of your business day. Do you see these people as negative, angry, non-talkative, and defensive in their daily interaction with you? Do you find people to be unfriendly or abusive in their dealings with people? Try to perceive the good traits in people. Try changing your perception, and focus on one positive feature within people. Bring out the positive qualities to the people themselves, because the people may not see the beauty of themselves. Compliment them. Find good truths to relate to them in a loving way.

We are energy and we function not only from our own energy but from the energy of other people that are interacting with our energy. If we see only the negative energy in other people, we are failing to accept the responsibility and strength of our own energy forces. Therefore, we allow the energy of others to control the energy of self. We must learn control of our own energy, which means that we must first accept that we are energy and matter. We must learn not to be controlled by the energy of others, which can have a disastrous effect on our lives and what we want to create.

Within every Soul there are good and honest virtues. Perceive the good. Focus on the positive. This will send them your energy of love. The negative energy of another person will be cancelled out by your positive energy. We can always overcome negative energy with positive energy. When we perceive the positive energy within ourselves, we will perceive the positive energy within our fellow human being. Within this perception is the miracle of love that has the power to heal all injuries.

If we were perfect, we would be living the Ethical Values of the Spirit. We would not be here on Earth. When we perceive ourselves in the negative sense, we are judging ourselves to be less perfect than we are. We are the problem, not the other person. Looking within ourselves and finding the positive energy of self will allow us to see only the positive energy in another. Changing our perception requires changing our belief system. In our belief system, there is right and wrong. Each perception is formulated by a conscious judgment of the right or wrong of the action. We can only perceive in judgment if we believe in the concept of right and wrong. There is no right, and there is no wrong. There is no judgment. There is the moment, the IS of Being.

If we can perceive the concept of right and wrong within the concept of time, it will be easier for us to understand the direct relationship of right or wrong to the issue of judgment, as dictated by time. For example, for many centuries we ate with our hands without benefit of utensils. When this occurred, it was judged right for the time. In the present moment of our time, it would be judged wrong if we picked up all of our food and ate it with our hands. Time changes our belief systems and therefore changes the entire concept of right and wrong within human logic. Time affects the judgment of right and wrong. Any concept that can be changed within a fleeting moment by our belief system cannot be part of the Universal Law of Spirit. The Law of Spirit is: "All things created by Spirit are eternal, and all things that are not created by Spirit are not real." Therefore, right and wrong and judgment are our belief system. They are not real, and they will change again in time as the belief system changes.

Within the Spirit world there is no time. There is no time on Earth. There is the illusion of time, which is created by our belief system for our own needs. Illusion, in the Spirit world, is defined as a false belief. We are incapable of making an honest judgment or truly conceiving of an honest assessment, because we cannot conceive of the reality of timelessness energy. Each Soul in the Universe is growing within its own growth pattern. This pattern is not governed by time because there is no time in the Spirit world. Time is a human creation. We created time in our need for structure. Our Soul IS where it must BE in its individual development. There is no right or wrong to the individual growth patterns, and our development, nor can there be any judgment of us and our growth. There is only the IS of the Now of all things within the Universe.

In the concept of our Earth time, there are Souls that are out of synchronicity with other cultures. They may act or speak in the context of the Soul culture in which they exist. That does not mean that we should judge them as wrong, because they fail to meet the standards of another person's belief system. They are true to their own being. Judgment is an ego acknowledgement, based on the belief in the rightness of our belief and the wrongness of the belief of our neighbor. It has no validity in reality. Judgment is an individual creation of negative energy, and has a direct energy impact only within the Dual Soul that created it.

Changing the need to judge anyone, by any standard, is a necessary step on the path to awareness. We cannot truly be aware of our own reality of self, if we are judging other Souls on Earth through our belief system. Giving up judgment is accepting self. It is allowing self, and all humans, to be self. It is embracing freedom. It is removing responsibility. There is endless freedom in not being required to judge. The freedom to accept self and our fellow human being, just as he is, removes a major conflict of ego and Soul from our physical reality. The path to awareness has been established and now it can be pursued with Love within us.

The Cycle of Awareness will begin in life in many ways and at different times. It is normal for us not to recognize what is happening in our world. Suddenly we find ourselves thinking, "I don't want to do this anymore." We may have problems identifying exactly what it is that we no longer want to do. This is the time to look within, at the *you* that you have created. For many, this will happen at a time when they are experiencing loss. It may be loss from physical death, separation of relationships such as children leaving home, dissolution of marriage, changes in professional positions, breaking up with someone we love, leaving a geographical area, or any number of changes that will require us to look at self, which can cause grief within us.

We identify with the physical world around us to such a degree that any loss is experienced with fear. This fear is the direct result of not loving self. Not recognizing the self, which is the Eternal Spirit and therefore inexhaustible, allows any loss to threaten the reality of the physical world as we see it. *Understand that true learning in our emotional health is Spiritual growth.* Experiencing Spiritual growth frees us from the fear and the loss that we experience in the physical sense. Changes in life are accepted as necessary and as part of Spiritual growth.

Without change, the Spirit is locked into the time frame of the physical.

The Spirit seeks change, growth and love. It cannot be static in time. The Spirit seeks oneness and accepts that all are one. In the physical sense we operate from the "I" concept. In our world we hear, "I did this, I bought this, I like this, I am, I, I, I, I, I." This is a self-centered, self-directed, self-focused, egotistical view of the world and our relationship to it. This "I" perception does not create change, indeed does not allow change, because the role of the "I," the ego, could not be maintained with change. We live in an ego-controlled world. Our reality is controlled by the ego of self, because the Spirit does not exist in the awareness of self. The Spirit has become overgrown with the struggle of the ego to maintain supremacy.

The need of the ego to control is our need to survive, in our mind. This is an illusion. If we know only one type of response to the world around us, and we are afraid of change, we are forced to protect what we see as SELF. Life for us is a daily battle for survival. It is *kill or be killed,* in the physical sense of our everyday reality. This concept of life is living in fear, and it is accepting and reinforcing the reality of fear, to self. Fear is accepted as such a necessary "survival emotion," that we create it as a necessary part of our daily existence. Without the benefit of awareness of the Soul and the Spirit of life as the balancing factor in the self that we have created, we are stuck with the ego and survival in the only terms known to the ego. As we develop awareness, we will be forced to deal with the ego and the fear that is created by the ego. This is the time of physical life when the ego and the Dual Soul reach their peak in conflict. The Soul is in a struggle for recognition and acknowledgement and the ego is in the struggle for survival. The Soul does not believe in struggle, but it recognizes that we must repeat what we do not learn. The Soul has an obligation to persist in its efforts to teach the ego balance.

The Soul sees the physical body and the mind under the control of the ego. The Soul sees us surviving in fear. This fear is equivalent to a heavy fog. When fear exists in our world, it affects our entire world. Fear does not stay in one little area of life, locked up in the special room and not allowed to come out. Fear surrounds, it permeates, and it becomes our "Consciousness." Fear is the fog in our life. Everything we experience in our physical life is judged by and decided upon from this created reality of fear. Our internal ego has used fear in its war with the mind and loving emotions through aeons of time in our life and evolution as human beings. Becoming aware of our fear and learning to release our fear is letting the Spirit of self out into world view. It is challenging the ego. It is saying, "I am me, I have the right to be me, I love me." It is recognition of our internal and eternal self. Acknowledging the Spirit self is equivalent to inflating the third tire of the super jet. Having that third tire fully inflated allows our super jet to speed down the runway, full of confidence in a safe and happy landing.

Awareness of the Spirit self is not destruction of the ego. The ego itself will undergo change from the influence of the Spirit, but they will not be able to be together productively. Awareness of the Spirit is the awareness of love. Love is the opposite emotion to fear. They cannot exist together. Love will envelop our world. It will permeate. It will heal. It will teach. It will BE us and our life. The shining white light of love will burn off any fog, no matter how thick it might be. As we enter this second cycle of life, we are searching for the love of self. We are searching for the awareness of love. We are searching for validation of our physical existence. We have been plagued with the thought, "Is this all there is to life?" We are judging life from the life that we have created from our belief system. We see a life of work, struggle, loss, and fleeting happiness. We see life as having an oasis, a place of Joy that we know exists but that we can't personally find. We are looking for that "something" missing in our life, but we simply don't know where it is nor do we understand clearly what it is. That oasis of joy is awareness of and love of self, our core self, or our Soul.

The Soul and Spirit of us are one, but they are separate. Our Soul is the memory of all experiences since the beginning of Soul creation. Our Spirit is the selected learned memories of the Soul that mirror the perfection of Spirit. These perfect images of Spirit that we have managed to learn in our overall Soul experience are in our memory. All experiences that the Dual Soul has lived from the beginning of Soul creation are part of the brain structure. Our Spirit is the selected learned memories of the Soul that mirror the perfection of Spirit and that exist as an energy of the brain. These images of Spirit that we have managed to learn have created our overall Soul experience and are separate as the Spirit of the Soul, yet they are one with the Soul and one with our hidden memories.

The Human is a trilocular design of energy as a body, mind and Spirit. The three are one and yet they are separate. Spirit is "the Father, the Son and the Holy Spirit." All That Is, is a trilogy of trilogies. No one can make us happy and joyful but us. We may seek wealth, work, play, religion and relationships, but none of them has the power to bring happiness and peace in the same way that knowledge can bring peace, joy, and happiness into our Heart and Soul and Spirit. Loving self, as the Spirit energy that we are, is the one way to find joy in living. It is also the way to find health in life. Without the joy and the awareness of the core self, we will not find the true self to love. Our focus will remain on the "I" of the ego, and we will continue in our life of fear and our consistent "fight" for survival.

Growing in awareness is learning to love the body, mind and Spirit of self. It is being in a world of love and health. It is functioning from the energies of the trilocular, integrated world of self as primarily an energy being. As we age, our belief system dictates that we begin the regression into second childhood. This belief system structures life as reaching a point where the rest of existence is a downhill slide to the bottom, or death. This must be one of the first changes that we make in our current belief system. If we continue to believe that we are reaching the point of regression, we will regress. Fortunately, for most of us this ego belief loses force with the advancing of life, and it remains more of a belief for the young than the old. This belief in eventual senility interferes with our ability to maintain awareness. This belief has filled our world with Souls that are so attached to physical matter they have failed to enter the Cycle of Awareness.

We gain the experience of Earth to deal with learning Earth lessons. If we fail to complete the lessons, the experience must be repeated in another incarnation. Our schools duplicate the school of life. If we do not complete the required courses, we understand that we will not receive the degree that we have been working on. Life is no different. When we see life as being all that has been and all that will be, we will not experience the restriction of Earth time. We will understand that growth and development are a continual process of living in physical lives. Life is more lenient and forgiving than any school that we have known. "Now" is the only moment of time that has validity for us on Earth, and life is being lived by the entire human species.

Developing an awareness of the inter-relatedness of the body, mind and Spirit will allow for the expansion of self with complete freedom. This is a concept that we have difficulty understanding totally. It requires opening up the mind and not judging. It requires a willingness to hear. It requires change. The physical self of body, mind, and Spirit is forever integrated, on Earth. It is the design of self that was created by Spirit. We do not appreciate, or use, the integration that has been given to us. For the most part we remain essentially unaware of the reality of the power which we possess, especially in our head and heart.

The Power of Experience

The inter-relatedness of the body, mind, and Spirit can be our saving grace, if we develop our awareness of the power that it creates. As we age, we are storing power through understanding, awareness, and knowledge of self, knowledge of the world, acknowledgement of the Universe and the emotions of love. This power is the power of experience, of knowing from the level of the Dual Soul, and it is absolute in its strength, which it allows us to live through the experience of controlling the reality of self.

Now, we have this understanding, this power that allows us to create our reality with control, with knowledge and with love. It is true that we are subject to the Law of Compensation, but understanding this allows retribution. That retribution is with self. If we are controlling self, that too is within our immediate and knowing control. As a physical, mental, and Spiritual being, at this time we are confronted with the integration of that physical and mental being. We know intuitively that the Spiritual being is safe. The Spiritual being is eternal.

We alone can take the step forward into the awareness of being and continue to be. We will need to evaluate the self from within. What does the self choose to do about life? The burden of senility is a lesson of the world. It is there for all of us to evaluate. What we live by, we will live through. We will become what we believe, without awareness. In the instances where this is a major lesson, it is an agreed upon lesson for all of those involved. There are Souls that know, from a Soul level, they will never choose a life of senility for themselves. They are aware Souls that understand the power and control that they have in creating their own consciousness and physical reality.

They have the understanding of body, mind awareness that gives them control. They have the understanding of mind and Soul awareness that will give them the right and freedom of choice. They will know when it is time for them to leave the Earth and they will leave. They will understand the completion of the purpose of the Soul in this Earth life. They will make either a conscious or subconscious choice, to make a transition for a new birth to continue learning their lessons with the choice of a new physical body. As human beings we live eternal life, which is a string of individual physical lives that we dedicate to learning through the lessons of each life.

We are learning to understand, by first understanding self, that all of life is a choice. This understanding allows each person the freedom to live with total and creative vitality, until the Dual Soul decides by conscious choice to leave Earth. But we must preserve our physical temple while on Earth. We cannot live as a human without having a home to live in. The senility that is common today is the Law of Compensation living out its effect in the energy of our human mind. We have failed to care for the physical body. We have failed to continue to develop into the Cycle of Awareness. Our physical body and our integrated self can continue to be in a healthy and productive state, as long as we respect, appreciate, and care for the development of our trilocular self, which is the physical body, thinking mind, and eternal Spirit as the true energies of the human species.

The way to begin this conscious creation is with the physical self, just as it was at the moment of birth. The physical self is the first and foremost part of self that must be cared for in the physical world. The physical self is subject to the Laws of Physical Matter. The physical self is the part of self that is the grounding of self as an energy being. It is the part that makes us human. We cannot and must not ignore our physical body at any point of our Earthly existence, if we want to stay within the physical realm. We must accept total responsibility for the condition of the physical. We cannot turn that responsibility over to physicians, family, friends, or caretakers. It is first and foremost our responsibility. We can accept guidance and assistance in caring for ourselves, but the primary responsibility belongs to us, at all points in our physical life. Caring for the physical will be covered in another chapter of this book. It will guide you in responsibly caring for your physical self.

The physical age of fifty years to one hundred years is the second season of life. It is the Cycle of Awareness. When we develop to the level of true balance within our energies, we will live to experience the two other seasons of our Earth life. For now, we will leave that explanation for another time. Developing awareness is the most exciting, creative gift that we can present to ourselves. It allows us to see the world with new eyes. It allows us to appreciate that which is new, that which is old, and that which is different. It broadens the perspective of life from a singular focus of self, to a multiple focus of All That Is. We have just entered the most creative and peaceful time of our life. Welcome it with Joy.

NATURE'S BALANCE
AS THE TRUTH OF HEALTH

Eating naturally of the foods from Nature is the perfect way for our society to give our physical body the food it needs for vibrant health. We are part of Nature. We need the foods of the Earth to support the health of our body, mind, and Spirit Consciousness. Processed food may once have known the Earth elements, but when we eat it, it has become a product of food and health pollution.

The research community of our medical world has seen and acknowledged that we do not eat in a manner that protects our body's health. We have been and are being told, by numerous sources, to change our diet to prevent disease. This need is only partially accepted by the medical community, and it is only partially accepted by everyone on Earth, but the purity of our foods, air, and water remains the primary method of creating good health and happiness with our life.

The foods that we have been given by our Creator are the foods of re-creation and restoration. When new mothers are carrying their unborn children, good diet is discussed and encouraged. After that one small outburst of wisdom from the Medical Community, they go "silent" and stop telling men, women, mothers or youth how to eat. The foods from a clean Nature are the best foods to eat for our health! We can add many years to each physical life simply by eating properly from the foods of Nature, plus breathing and drinking from the air and water of Nature. We could change our lifespan dramatically if we learned the true difference between organic foods and non-organic foods and ate accordingly to protect both our human body and our thinking mind.

We must eat the foods of Nature if we want to live our health and prevent disease. They are the foods of perfect digestion, assimilation and elimination. When they are utilized with the water and air of the Earth, there are no other needs of the physical body that are not being satisfied. Using the foods of Nature assures us that cellular viability is being maintained within our cellular body. This in turn assures us that the physical body will function as it was meant to function, with no excess waste material to create blockage and disease. Eating, drinking, and breathing from a clean Nature is our personal responsibility as human beings if we want to live without disease.

The foods of Nature create a cellular rhythm of energy within our body that protects and cleanses as it restores. A *feeling-tone* is created with this balanced cellular energy that allows us to open to the creative senses that have been bestowed by past understandings and Soul memories. This feeling-tone can join in the Universal energy fields, to reach its maximum in creativity and Joy.

This is the joy of health that can be the reality that we create for all people on Earth, when we totally understand the truth of our human relationship to Nature.

What is, in our world, is our creation for the sake of financial gain. The industrialization, commercialization and materialization of Earth has fashioned us into a pawn of a burgeoning commerce of supply and demand that can create good foods, but for the sake of money it creates many foods that are not especially healthy for most people. An eternal life lesson is found in the foods that we eat. Are we living ancient behaviors from our past lives? Are we lazy now and we do not want to exert our human body to grow natural organic foods? Business in this sense of chemically forced food production is financially productive for many, and physically destructive to the masses. The secret to life is that each and every person has free choice in what they select to buy and to eat. If we want to protect ourselves from the agony of disease, we must pay attention to the chemicals that we put into our human body. Many times we can be more certain of what we eat by growing what we eat. This is a viable choice. Because I grew up on a farm before the advent of chemicals, I did eat well and I learned the lesson well. Now I eat only organic foods.

The vibrational energy (feeling-tone) of big business in our world is not a productive energy force but instead it is a negative field of non-caring, ego-focused, unaware Souls, who in their concern for the financial realities bring about even their own physical destruction. This lack of awareness and understanding of exactly what their contribution is to the masses allows them the comfort of their ego focus until they too die. Financial success in our world is more creative when it does not injure those who support it so willingly. This can be, if it is done with Soul awareness that protects rather than destroys. Financial success that is the result of a recognized and acknowledged commitment to the welfare of humankind, and where the actions bring about only committed reactions, is a true Soul lesson. This is the creation of abundance that is secondary to the benefit of the service to humankind. Our system functions from what we call supply and demand. On the Spiritual plane that is known as action and reaction. Business provides what the world seeks. From this concept, the world is in control if they exercise their individual right of choice. This choice has created our world today.

The reality of our world today will be our early destruction in each incarnation and eventual destruction of Earth as we know it, without changes occurring in our belief system. This is the direct result of our actions reaching extreme proportions of greed. This is our ego that is no longer controlled by the total, balanced self. Destruction is not a Universal need nor is anything in our world pre-determined. Our events are created, just as our physical world is created, by us both individually and in mass. What we experience on Earth, we have created on Earth.

As an example, it has been understood in the scientific community for many years, that we are creating disease and death by the simple necessary action of eating. Our government has spent many hours researching this reality, just as others have. It is time for each individual to change the quality of food that they are choosing to eat. Both the organic foods and non-organic foods are sold today in the marketplace. We can protect ourselves and give ourselves a happier and healthier lifestyle that will help us live for many more years of life. This knowledge has not brought about significant change in Universal eating habits. It has created some change in those who are aware, but it has not created a change for the masses. Creating a change for the masses would interfere in the supply and demand levels that have currently been established. This in turn would create some degree of financial concern, for a short period of time, but once the adjustments were made to our food sources, everything would again balance out. A change in the way that we eat, think and live is the change that is necessary, if we are to be the most that we can be. Causing our own physical destruction and the destruction of our world as we know it will certainly not be productive for our species now or in future generations.

We must create a balance through the economic balance of supply and demand, before the masses of people on Earth will hear the danger of their current existence. The primary danger lies in the financial destruction of our world, which will impact on the lives of each and every human. A healthy person is a creative person that can find a solution to any problem. Eating from a clean Nature is paramount to the human population living as healthy human beings.

The habits that remove us from the energies of Earth also remove us from the energies of the Universal Mind and the energies of the Spiritual Universe. Our present economy has been created on our removal from the energies of Nature. This creates a change in us and in Earth. A significant volume of information is available to the masses from the Internet, books, magazines, newspapers, television and radio as our physical intellectual resources continue to expand. Some of this knowledge is creative for us but the majority of this information is surrounded by negative energy, which has a negative influence on all humans. It does not teach us how to think and live in a positive manner, or how to increase the life span of our physical body by the foods that we eat. Interest in the quality of one's life must be an individual choice and an individual understanding. Advertisements are misleading in their references to health. This is in many instances an innocent misrepresentation, but it is a misrepresentation (lie) even when done from a lack of awareness. The more we use drugs to support disease, the more money the drug czars make. When we eat correctly from the purity of Nature, we will remain healthy for a much longer period of time, and we will maintain our youth and vitality into old age.

As human beings, in general, we do not know that we are destroying our physical credibility. We live with a warm sense of safety, security and conformity within the world that we think we know and understand. We do not recognize or accept that the food we eat makes our physical body what it is. The concept that our daily eating habits are slowly and surely presenting true physical blockage in different systems of our body by the resulting residue or waste material is not part of our reality. Even more difficult for most people to understand is that we are chemical beings, and we must eat those chemicals that our body is using up by living. The harder we work, the more we need good foods.

Our mentality that "all food is good food" is destructive to the cellular structure and function of our physical self. This concept that all food is good food has allowed food processors to produce what tastes good to our addictive senses. The fats, sugars and starches that are the primary ingredients in processed foods are addictive and destructive to our cellular design because they do not give us the true nutrients from foods that are very important to our health and our happiness.

The eating habits of our world are so truly destructive that the results have created large industries to support the destruction of the physical self. These businesses are the drug companies, hospitals and nursing homes that absorb a large portion of the world economy as we recognize it. These businesses are parasitic to the diseases within us on Earth. They in turn cause more destruction. This cycle can only be changed by our increased awareness that we can live much longer than we are living if we keep our cells balanced internally.

How to become healthy: Happiness is taking charge of your health.

Loving our physical temple means that we feed it from Nature. Learn to eat the raw fruits and vegetables that your body was designed to thrive on, to stay young on, and to stay disease-free on. Eat only organically grown fresh foods. Eat some meats if your body craves them, but make certain that you buy them fresh from an organically aware farmer who has allowed his animals to graze on freshly grown organic pastures and to eat only pure food.

A recent incarnation of an advanced Soul spent his life learning Earth lessons, and sharing them with the world. He showed, by his own health example, that eating the foods of Nature can cure disease. His lesson was good for the world. He lived his life trying to convince the world that improper food intake creates disease. He reached many. A large percentage of his followers are advanced Souls in the world today. His name was Nathan

Pritikin. Many continue to read his books and believe in his words. In believing many will also change and do. This truly advanced Soul left a nutritional lesson for the world. We should listen.

We all will choose to leave our Earth incarnations when we feel that we have learned all that we can learn. Our last lesson in each lifetime is our death. Our way of transition to the Spiritual plane is chosen for reasons that may not seem related to the life that we have lived. Understand that the lesson of transition is as important as the lessons of living. Learning not to judge is another lesson of Earth life. Learn to observe with discernment. Be aware without judgment. Learning not to judge is an Earth lesson that takes us one step closer to our goal of perfection. Awareness gives us the freedom of individual choice without judgment.

Our society has become an "accepting" society, yet it does not want to accept the responsibility for personal health or personal disease. We must accept responsibility for self. There is no other way for us to live. Each of us is responsible for what we are and for what we eat. Allowing others to be responsible for our health, such as fast-food chains, food processors, the medical community and drug companies, is flirting with total degeneration of the physical self. We create our own reality. The responsibility for individual health belongs to the individual. The choice is ours. Blindly following the path of advertisements, fads, belief systems or any teacher without evaluating how it feels to us on an energy level is seeking problems. We are seeking our own individual balance of cellular energy. We must first know ourselves and the needs of our physical self to find the energy level that is perfect for us. It is a personal search. In a world of leaders, many have become followers.

The commercial mentality "All food is good food" has been taught in medical schools, nutrition programs and to the general public. Look at our health problems and we can observe that the concept, the belief, is not valid. Read the available research yourself. Choose your own belief. Raise your awareness level. Challenge yourself to learn all there is to learn about health and your body. Read with discernment because the challenge is in finding what truly works. In a world of leaders too many of us have made the conscious choice to follow others in the world of nutrition, despite the creativity that we exercise in other areas of our existence. There is joy and satisfaction in learning about our physical response to eating. There is joy and satisfaction in preparing and sharing good food with friends and family. There is complete cellular joy and happiness in feeling true vitality within. *When you eat something, how do you feel?*

The foods of Nature eaten in their natural state change our cellular energy. The time period required for this change will depend on the amount of waste material that is presently within our physical systems. When we are actively working to find this energy balance, we will instinctively know when we reach our balance. Our cellular energy will flow smoothly without waste matter, and we will physically feel a sense of lightness and health. Mentally we will feel a sense of happiness and joy, which may be totally foreign to us. We will find ourselves being more creative with our five physical senses, and with the Universal senses of our mind and Spirit. We will have reached our balance of the physical self.

Let the beginning of change for each of us be in forgiving ourselves. Feel no guilt for what you see as your past. It is not important what you have done. It is not important if you were an addict of some substance. Accept the choice of personal responsibility for the present moment, the *now* of life. Eating from Nature's food takes less time than anything else that we can do. Earth is an advanced world where we have access to the freshest fruits, vegetables, nuts, grains and seeds available in the world. Use these foods to your health advantage. Choose to make your eating experience an adventure in your life and eat organically whenever possible.

Some food producers and processors are becoming enlightened, and they truly want to keep their foods acceptable to the health conscious Soul. Their foods will be free of chemicals and preservatives. They will rely on the natural quality of the food and not add sugars, starches and fats to pollute the quality of nutrients. Fresh foods are always the foods of choice, but be aware that unpolluted foods must be searched out. These prepared foods should be used only as an occasional substitute for the fresh foods that our body truly needs. Never fail to read the labels of the processed foods that you purchase. We are truly unaware of what we eat.

Food pollution is common to preserve food and give it a longer shelf life, and consequently a longer opportunity to sell. This food is created for profit, not quality. Food pollution is destructive to our physical energy system and it frequently comes from unhealthy sources. It is the basis of disease and eventual death for many people. Food pollution does not consist of only the chemicals and preservatives that are used, but it also includes the fats, sugars and starches that are added to create the exact taste that we are now addicted to.

This preservation process can produce a de-mineralized, de-vitaminized, and polluted product that is dangerous to us. The waste material accumulates and nothing is then eaten to free this foreign matter from the physical systems. Processed food is a study in excesses and deficiencies. The quality of the food that is eaten can be seen in the percentage of our population that suffers from indigestion and constipation and routinely uses drugs for heartburn and laxatives. Laxatives in our society are a "best-seller" for the drug companies, as are anti-acids. *Learn to support your own health first, rather than supporting drug companies.*

The human body is made to digest, assimilate, and eliminate waste food. If we are eating from the foods of Nature and drinking pure water, this is a natural process. With the use of a simple steamer we can have a delicious meal fresh from Nature's bounty. Our food intake should consist of three to six fresh fruits a day and four to eight fresh or steamed vegetables a day. These foods will energize and cleanse the body of waste material. In the beginning of our balancing process, we should not consume the second generation foods of Nature. The exact method and foods that can be used for this process will be outlined in another area of this book.

Eating truly from the foods of Nature will not require us to have a concern about the calorie consumption that is still our primary focus today. Health is an eating adventure. We need to eat to restore our cells. Our concern should be for the quality of the foods that we eat, and their relationship to their natural state. We were made from soil to live from the soil. It is the soil and the foods that grow from the soil that maintain the chemical cellular viability in the plant foods and in our human body. Until we, as human beings, can learn to maintain cellular viability we will be unable to live a longer life of good quality, because our chemical imbalance will create diseases, especially cancer.

We should never feel safe and comfortable in our attempt to replace the nutrients of the soil from today's vitamin and mineral preparations. The digestion, assimilation, and elimination of these products will vary from person to person, based upon many other circumstances. Reliance on artificial replacements is a false sense of security for any physical Soul. Using these preparations for short periods of time is occasionally beneficial but not as efficient to the cellular structure as the foods of Nature would be. Supplements are not capable of maintaining cellular viability over long periods of time. They are treated as foreign matter by the body and can present their own ravages to the cellular structure. Believing that these substances can replace eating is an illusion. It is not within the Law of Nature.

The very creation of being a physical being dictates that we must exist in a physical body. Our physical body is only one component of self. It is the clearly defined physical temple of the Spirit. Our total self consists of three component parts – BODY, MIND, and SPIRIT. This is an Earth reality, not to be forgotten. We must clearly understand or we will not see the value in balancing the physical self through these three component parts. One part does not work well without the other two parts, which is the primary reason that people are now facing a choice of learning in a forward motion or back-sliding into our fears.

Much has been said about the role of the Spirit in our total self, by the churches and the scribes of history. The Spirit has had a lot of press in our world, from the focus of religion. This concept of our Spirit has not always been Spiritual. Our society has focused for many years on the component of self that we call the mind. This focus has been on the singular part of the mind that is the intellectual mind, with some appreciation for the rational mind. Until recently in our society there has been only small concern for the intuitive mind. There has been extreme distrust of any perspective of abilities that may exist outside of the physical senses. Of course this is our internal response to fear as a reflection of our belief systems.

The physical self has not known a balanced focus on Earth since 1500 AD. It was during this period that man began to deny the relationship of himself as part of Nature. Through the years the human has moved further and further from that sense of reality, and has viewed the body as a societal appendage rather than an integrated part of the total self. The physical self has become as a leaf on a tree. It is abused and ravaged by every new concept that blows through our world. It is dictated to by society, rather than by Nature. It is forced to conform to a belief system that fails to see the physical self in its true role of eternal growth. We believe that the body is separate from the mind and Spirit, and must be a product of our culture to be appreciated. Physical acceptance now depends on the right shape, the right accessories, the right makeup and the right hairstyle. These are the beliefs of struggling Souls. The lesson of the physical is the lesson of integration. You are not five-feet-two with eyes of blue.

That is a physical perception of the beholder that does not yet understand energy and its power within the human being. The physical is an illusion. As physical matter we are all unique, and it does not work to try to mold our body into a stereotypical physical image. Within each body there is the perfect balance. This balance is an energy of life and it will be known by the physical joy that we feel when we reach this balance. We will understand it in the health that we enjoy. It cannot be measured by the vision of society, but only by the reality of true cellular function. Only you can truly seek the balance of your physical self. Only you can truthfully live the balance of your energy self and learn to grow from within your internal energy.

Some questions to ask of yourself for guidance are: Do you feel well? Are you free of dis-ease and disease? Are you strong and active? Do you have energy and motivation for living? Do you always speak and live your truth? Do you choose to use your thinking mind as your level of growth and change? Do you feel within yourself the joy of physical health? Do you like yourself? Are there any substances that you use excessively in your life? Do you abuse your body with indiscriminate sexual activity? Do you exercise daily? Do you sincerely try to eat the foods of Nature whenever possible? Do you drink plenty of water?

All answers should be yes, with the exception of two. If you answered in this way, you are trying to live a balanced life. Balance is measured in multiple degrees of energy. Try to be the best that you can be physically, mentally and Spiritually. Each part of self can be evaluated in the same way. When each part of us is in perfect balance, the unity will happen. Do not live with the illusion that we can function from one part of self and not the other parts of self, and find our true balance. True balance encourages enlightenment and Soul evolution. True balance must be reached before true attunement can be experienced. Many people believe they can reach a certain type of "Nirvana" through other people. This is an illusion. We are responsible for our own growth, which we can encourage by expanding our thinking mind, loving emotions, and our Spirit Senses. None of these growth experiences will be apparent, nor can they be judged by our physical appearance. They will be seen in the way we live, the things we do, the people that we are, and most of all they will be clearly reflected through our interaction with other people. Our energies will be experienced by others in the energy essence of peace and love that will surround us, if and when we can open our thinking mind to the understanding of energy within us.

The health of the thinking mind is essential to this integration of our physical body with our Dual Soul and our Spirit Consciousness Energies. Health of the mind is in itself a separate integration just as the body and Spirit are separate integrations. The thinking mind cannot function totally from the intellectual mind because it must be a balance of rational, intellectual, and intuitive thought processes that are interacting together to create logic and understanding within us in relationship to our external image of ourselves.

The thinking mind requires freedom and openness. It cannot be controlled by the ego self or a belief system and still continue to function openly. For health, the thinking mind must be non-judgmental, loving, sharing, open, trusting, truthful, faithful, and aware. It must be allowed that balance that gives it creativity and joy. It must value itself and be love in action. The Spirit too must have a balance. It must be coordinated with the actions of the thinking mind just as the body is coordinated with the actions of the thinking mind. A healthy mind will help assure us of a healthy Spirit Consciousness because the reflection is there in the thinking and reactions of our intellectual mind. Balancing the Spirit Consciousness is knowing the love of self, of the Spirit self, and of thy neighbor, as one integrated energy field. The knowledge of our total love, truth, and perfection is the total balance of our internal Spirit Consciousness. There is no other way.

These are the balances that Nature seeks in the total self of the human being. Begin with the body, add the thinking mind and the Spirit to create an energy that is easier to understand and explore. See and accept your life as the adventure that it is. Do not fear change. Invite it into your world. Take risks. Be open and joyful. Be the love that you are, within the perfection of your Spirit Consciousness that is motivating you to be the very best that you can be. Jealousy always destroys love. This is a major issue between lovers, marriages, and friends. We can never live jealousy and love at the same time in our physical lives because the two energies that are involved in jealousy and love are diametrically opposite and therefore they never function together. If we are harboring jealousy, it affects us but it does not affect the person that we are feeling jealous of or loving towards. Our emotions are individualistic to us and cannot be shared by another person.

Our society has a saying that "love is blind." Love is aware. Man is blind. Love sees the true essence of the physical. Love sees the integration of the body, mind, and Spirit. Love sees energy. As physical matter we are energy, as mind we are energy, as Spirit we are energy. Energy manifests in the physical world as light. Imagine yourself as a shining white light. You are now seeing the energy of self as you are using your energy. If you look and you see nothing new, you are restricting your own internal energy flow.

It is the thinking mind that sees the physical energy in each of us. It is the thinking mind, and the belief system that it is controlled by, that judges man in the physical concepts of living his life. Each person is and should be as unique in the physical self, as we are in the Dual Soul and Spirit Consciousness. The thinking mind and our loving emotions are the structure of our Dual Soul. We frequently want to create clones of ourselves, of the physical image of our belief system. There is no acceptance of individuality in the thinking mind of most people. There is little appreciation of the uniqueness of self, especially within the thinking mind, loving emotions, and Spirit Senses.

Our Dual Soul's gradual evolution to an integrated state allows for the crystal clear vision of true physical energy on a Spiritual level. The need to balance the physical self is the need to balance the total energetic self. Our thinking mind, loving emotions, and Spirit senses cannot be balanced if the physical self is not balanced. Balancing the total self is living our evolution of the integration of self. Balancing the total self is the gift of freedom for the body, mind and Spirit. Because we are basically energy at our core, in all parts of ourselves, we must balance the energies in our various parts before we can feel any sense of balance in our physical lives.

We are designed with an inner peace.

Freedom of the thinking mind allows the chains of our previous belief systems to dissolve from our present physical reality and allows us to live our absolute freedom of choice. We are designed with an inner peace. Peace is the result of accepting the unity of self, the perfection of self, and the love of the Spirit Self. Our Dual Soul has found the understanding of oneness within in relationship to the physical body and the Spirit Consciousness. The blockage of any one component part of the total self will interfere with the balance of the integrated whole. We cannot deny the body and be balanced within our mind. We cannot deny the integrated mind and be balanced in the physical body. We cannot deny Spirit and be balanced in our eternal energy. There is no other way.

Our Energy Balance is not for another person to judge, but it will be observed in the actions of joy and inner peace or our anger and fear. It will be known and cherished by the Dual Soul who is reaching this level of integration. The energy blockages, if they occur, will be consciously removed by the Dual Soul. They will be examined, reconstructed, and understood. This action will always be guided by our Spirit Consciousness. These are always internal changes, and they are found within the total energy self. The internal actions may or may not manifest external changes, which will not matter. *Changing the energy that we use within our human body is the primary issue.* An example of dramatic change is when a person has become a chronic liar which is used as a means of self-protection. Once the person can understand that lying is getting in their way of friendships, they will be willing to change. Many people use lying as a means of bolstering the ego, which reveals volumes about their state of thinking in the mind.

Traveling through life as an enlightened Soul requires that we continually seek our individual balance.

That balance is not out there floating in the Universe; it is within the total self of us as Earth creatures. We create our world, our health, our experiences, our lives, and our attitude about life and living. Everything that we experience is a lesson to assist with that overall state of internal balance that we are striving to maintain. There is no wrong. There is no blame. What is has to be for the sake of learning our internal balance. You are precisely where you have grown into as your own personal physical creation is happening. You are responsible for who you are and no one can change you, but you.

The energy balance that each person is seeking can best be found in the rhythm of Nature. Returning to that rhythm in the things that we do, the foods that we eat, the sounds that we enjoy, the smells that refresh us, the air that restores us, and the water that soothes us, is the way of seeking Nature's balance in our own Earthly existence.

KATHY ODDENINO

NUTRITION FOR RESTORATION AND HEALTH

To understand the nutrition that is essential for the physical body, we need to understand the relationship of the physical body to the thinking mind, loving emotions, and the Spirit Consciousness, and we must see these three parts of ourselves as an energy of Earth, Nature, and Air. As physical bodies we are energy and all parts of us are energy. The chemical energy of our cellular structure supplies us with the overall energy to be in human form.

Our thinking mind is the builder of our internal cellular energy. Our thinking mind chooses the food that we eat and the activity that we involve our physical bodies in to help us grow and change. Once that choice is made by the thinking mind, the body responds by eating and by physical activity. *The mind is the builder, the body is the result.* Hold this statement mentally with you as you continue reading this chapter, because this is the delineation of responsibility in the world, which each and every person must learn to understand. Knowing that we do indeed create what we need, including the presence of disease, can present us with another choice to make. If we aren't healthy, we must ask, why am I not healthy?

Are we choosing our foods wisely? Food and water show us our choice as the choice of health. Today the foods that are eaten are no longer pure in Nature, which allows cancer and other diseases to run rampant in and through the human species. *We have within us three types of energy.* Earth energy is the cellular energy of the physical body. Earth energy is the energy from the Earth elements themselves. The energy that is restored within the self from the utilization of the air, the water, and the plant foods of Nature gives us health. When the Earth energy is balanced within the physical self, it will magnetize additional Earth energy from the ground to provide you with extra energy grounding, which will keep you physically balanced as a human being.

Universal energy, which is the energy of the mind, is available from the Universe in vast quantities even when it is not being used to its maximum. Universal energy is the energy of Universal knowledge. All that is or will be has been. The energy of this knowledge is there, within the Universe, for all of us to draw upon. Spiritual energy is the energy of the true Spirit self within us. Spiritual energy is inexhaustible, if we acknowledge and use it in our daily living. Spiritual energy is the Spirit energy. It is the motivation of life, it is our Spirit Consciousness.

The Energy of the mind and Spirit are easier to balance, and therefore use, when the physical energy is balanced. An example of this energy drain can be seen in addiction, especially with drugs or alcohol. This is a very unbalanced energy that is draining to other people and to the mind and Spirit of the Soul involved. Looking at our world from an energy perspective, this is shown by the tremendous amount of energy that is focused by millions of people towards their dis-ease and disease. As human beings, we expect to have disease. This is a negative, or draining energy for the mind and Spirit. The physical self is so far off balance that the mind and Spirit of self become lost in the depths of the negative energy.

Recognizing the importance of the physical energy and what it can do for us on all three planes makes the choice of caring for the physical body more important. The physical body is our point of power in the physical world. Treat the needs of your physical body with respect. Do not abuse it and it will serve you well. Understanding that it is our thinking mind that makes us what we are physically gives us the freedom to create what we want and desire in our physical world. Do we truly want diseases such as cancer, AIDS, herpes, arthritis, multiple sclerosis, and a host of other diseases? I think not, for most of us.

Know that disease or health can both be our choice. Our reaction to the action of our mind has created a physical imbalance within and exposed us to disease. We create the reality of our health, in the same way that we create the reality of the rest of our world. Accepting the responsibility for our actions is the first step in being what we want to be. We create the lessons of life in many ways, but the primary way is thinking without any consideration for the thoughts we are choosing, and the secondary way is exposing our human body to chemicals that are not healthy for us.

Creating our lessons as disease means on a Spiritual level that we refuse to deal with an issue directly on a physical level. When we refuse to deal with our lessons then we must keep repeating them. Disease is a method of aborting the life design. It can also be used to remind ourselves of the life plan, and it can be used to get our attention directed back to the life plan and the intention for us to learn. Lessons are more interesting when they can be worked out as dramas of joy, which are the perfect dramas of life. Life shows us the way of the perfect lesson and it is something to strive for in our world. In a drama of Joy the lessons will occur with as much impact but with less drama and trauma.

The significance of the lessons of the Soul will usually be more profound. The issue can be understood more clearly from the state of health than the state of trauma or disease. There are physical laws that we must be subjected to with trauma that create dramas within dramas. One of the most important lessons for the human being is the lesson of Nutrition. Eating nutritionally to help us live vitally comes from all three energy sources of Earth, Universe and Spirit. It is available to us all equally. We all have the same capabilities. We are all equal as human beings. We do not all have the same level of awareness, so we do not use the energy from all three sources equally. It is there for us when we open to its presence.

Despite the questionable condition of our physical self at this moment in time, it can be restored to a large degree if our mind is willing and our intention is strong. We cannot take away chronological age but we can take away many of the ravages of physical abuse, if we are willing to make that commitment to our physical self. When we commit our thinking mind to restore and revitalize our basic cellular structure, our physical self will respond if we act on that commitment. Until there is the commitment of the mind, the intent and the will of action will not work efficiently. A commitment of the mind will require drinking and eating Nature's foods for the Earth energy supply to be at its maximum to assure proper digestion. We will need to keep the body active, so that assimilation and elimination will function properly. Choose friends wisely and find comfort in their presence.

These activities will relieve us of dis-ease and disease to create a new physical self. This change will also benefit the restoration of the endocrine system, where the energy blocks normally occur to the Spiritual energy of self. People with disease or dysfunction of the endocrine system are consciously blocking their Spiritual energy on an unconscious physical level. The beginning of relinquishment of all energies is the commitment of the mind to strengthen the physical energies of self.

Once this commitment is made, the first step to action is a change in our thinking, eating habits and our activity level. This will seem to be a monumental task for some. If so, they need to continue working on this decision, from a mind level. The commitment has not been made. When we can truthfully say, "I am in control of my physical self" and know it to be true, we are ready to proceed. Think only in terms of the "you" you want to BE. Visualize the You of your dreams and imagination. Let this image become so strong that it remains consistently within your psychic, or third eye vision. This vision is your unconscious vision that occurs in the middle of your forehead, not within your physical eyes. This is your Spiritual vision. With consistent imaging you will see it as real in the physical world. This is your blueprint. This is your pattern for building a new physical body and a new thinking mind.

It is vital to have this blueprint clearly envisioned to constantly refer to, in your work of restoration. Your mind is in the process of building a new you. It needs a pattern. If we were going to build a house, we would first have an architect draw us up a set of blueprints. We would take this pattern, this design, and we would start building. When we begin to build and restore the body to health we are the architect. We draw the blueprint as we want to be and then we set about the task of building. We will respond to what our mind has created, so know that you are creating the perfect self. Let your imagination search until you have that perfect image defined and photographed clearly within your memory cells. It must be you. The perfect you.

We cannot create, for instance, a self that does not need to stay in balance with the Laws of Nature. *Our mind will not create an unrealistic image.* What we have in our mind will be what we create. It is helpful to find a picture of yourself, when you looked as you would like to look now. Put it in a place of frequent vision. This will help you with your blueprint. If you would like to be even better than the picture, make these adjustments mentally each time that you look at the picture. When the vision is firm in your mind, remove the picture.

At this time we must also surround ourself with the protection of our Spiritual energy. This will keep our body from being influenced by the temptations and comments of our wishful mind. Envision an envelope of pure white light surrounding you, over your head and under your feet. This is an unbroken energy force. Request that it protect you from all temptation. This is your Spiritual shield. Other people's judgments of you will not be able to penetrate this energy shield. You are peaceful and serene within. You are building. You are creating. Negative influences are a basic problem, when any Soul on the physical level decides to make changes. We leave ourselves vulnerable to the judgments of others.

We are intent on conforming to beliefs, and in our belief that we are right we are persistent in our need to have others conform. This validates our belief system, as being right within our world. These people do not like change, they do not believe in change, and they will resist change in other people as creatively as they resist change in themselves. Request that they be in peace and joy, but keep your commitment to yourself. Your Spiritual shield will protect you. Having made the commitment in our mind to protect our cellular structure, we must make a commitment to protect the physical self from the outside energy forces. It is within our control. It is our individual choice.

Changing our lifestyle is a positive approach to changing our eating habits and activity habits. Those influences in our life that are creating negative energy must be dropped from our reality. These negative forces can be identified, if they remove our freedom to be ourselves and if they restrict the Joy within us. Turn them loose, let them go. Thank them from your Spirit, for having contributed to the evolution of your Soul, and say goodbye. If you spend a few hours of mental evaluation of your lifestyle, your thoughts and your actions, the parts of your life that are not working for you will become apparent.

This exercise is not to make anyone in our world wrong. It is to face the reality of our own self. It is looking at our world, to see where we find joy and happiness. The activities in our world that give us happiness and joy or allow us to be happy and joyful are the activities to continue. Do not expose yourself any longer to activities or people that are needy and draining for you. This must be our choice, if we have made our commitment to health. Health is JOY. Joy is Love. For many of us this new awareness may require that we look intently at our business world. If we cannot function in our work with joy and happiness, it is not right for us if we want to be a whole and healthy person. Do what you love to do in life. We have a choice to be in an energy vampire situation or to be in peace and joy. All of life is a choice.

Once the mind has developed the image of self that will lead you to the Joy of Health, and it has filtered out those energy forces that are draining you, it is time to begin the restoration of your physical body. You are now joyful in your environment, and it is time to turn your focus to your physical body. Your image of the perfect self is in place. Your physical body is a structural unit and a functioning unit. You must maintain the structure and the function to enjoy the living. This book is not intended as a textbook on anatomy, but to explain the body's need for Nature's food it is necessary to touch briefly on the structure of the physical self.

Our One Basic Responsibility

The physical body, which appears in physical matter as one unit, is composed of billions of units on the cellular level. These cells join together to form tissues, organs, systems, bones, blood and many other structures, within various structures. Each has its own integrity, but each works as a part of the total. This unity provides perfect function, if the basic cellular integrity is not challenged. The cellular formation within the physical body provides the architectural image of self, the structure, and the artistic image of self, the function.

Compromising even one group of cells in our body puts the total body structure and function at risk. The primary function of the body is survival. It does survive with amazing efficiency, despite the consistent insults that we provide it in the living. If the function of the body depends on the credibility of the smallest of cells, we need to understand how that tiny cell maintains its credibility. The body has many different types of cells, and some of the requirements vary, but we are going to speak to these as a total. Cellular integrity requires oxygen, water, protein, fat, carbohydrates and organic mineral salts, which are all part of plant material. Therefore, we can truly say that in order to maintain our human cellular integrity we need only oxygen, water and plant material.

All of the physical requirements of the body are Earth elements. If these elements are provided, with the plant material being provided in variety, the body will maintain cellular viability. The structure of the cells determines the function of the cells. What we give the body for the structure of the cells will determine how the total body functions. There is no other way. The responsibility that has been given to us is a simple one. The activity of the cells is a complex integration that depends upon digestion, assimilation, and elimination within the physical body. *We do not have to worry about the cellular activity, as long as we fulfill our one basic responsibility.*

We must supply the elements of Nature that restore and maintain the viability of the cellular structure and function of our physical body. Cellular function is totally complex and is programmed into each individual cell. We can take the cellular function for granted and give it no thought, if we fulfill our responsibility. Cellular function is intensely fascinating because it is better at "making do" with what we provide than anyone can ever duplicate. The physical body was given to us as a temple, by our human creation as a miracle of Spirit. We are the energy, the essence of Spirit. That is our true identity. We are the Spirit self, we are HU-MAN. We are a Higher Universal MANA.

We will never totally unravel the complexities of the Universe of the human body, but we will continue to accept it as our challenge even when we do not understand what we have discovered and how to use it successfully. We have approached this challenge from the mechanistic, scientific approach and the emotional and Spiritual approach. The physical self is not either/or. One part of our human design does not work without the other. The body constantly shows us the results of its mind and its heart. It reminds us of the physical sensory reality by giving us pain and disease, when we fail to maintain its cellular integrity. The commercial mentality of our world is allowing us to deny our individual responsibility for our cellular function. We feel our body will always be fixable – not by Spirit, the Master Designer, but by man, the creation of the True Architect.

This is the path of taking from the Spirit self, and giving to the unknown. It is a path of refusing to accept responsibility for self. It is a path of deterioration and pain. We live in a world of commercialization. We have an advanced Earth. Commercialization is a world that leads us away from the world of Nature, where we must restore the elements of our body. We have become a society of fast food addicts. Fast food does little to maintain cellular viability. It contributes greatly to the waste material that is the source of many of our diseases. When we eat food of little natural value, we have no desire to eat the foods of Nature. We become satisfied. Our hunger is appeased with lots of fat and lots of sugar. We have also invited a host of reactions for our physical self to manage. These foods are inadequate to maintain consistent health of our physical body. How can we be healthy?

With very little thought, we can purchase the freshest fruits, vegetables, nuts, grains and seeds available. These are the first foods that were provided for us. They are the first generation foods. These foods contain the elements of Nature that will maintain our cellular structure. They are our building materials. We can create beautiful meals that will satisfy and energize the physical self, from the foods of the Earth. Foods such as meat, fish, chicken, and all foods of the flesh are second generation foods. These are foods that have themselves been created and survive by the plants of Nature. Third generation foods are those produced by the Second generation foods such as milk, eggs, and honey.

None of these foods are wrong. The damage to the physical body is committed by the excesses and deficiencies of the food that we eat. We have a habit of eating to excess. We eat what we like and we resist change. We eat what tastes good, not what is good for us. We eat very little variety. We eat the same thing day in and day out from habit. An example of eating practices that are harmful to the integrity of the physical self is the large consumption of red meat. Many times meat is consumed to the exclusion of the other foods of Nature. Red meat has no fiber, it is high in fat, and it has little if any organic mineral salts by the time that it is consumed. Antibiotics, hormones, and other chemicals given to the animals have increased the contaminants we ingest when we eat a lot of "commercial" meat. Meat is usually accompanied by potatoes, corn, bread, beer and pie or cake in our culture. This menu will practically guarantee us a significant bout with indigestion and perhaps an episode of "gout."

This is a meal of fat, starch and sugar. These are all acid-producing foods within our body. There will also be a tendency to eat quickly and chew our food only briefly. By not chewing we did not start the digestive process with the mastication of food with saliva. Chewing would have provided some alkalinity to the meal. Now the food is in our stomach, where the hydrochloric acid is being diluted by the beer. It does not digest. It remains in the stomach and the acid foods start to ferment. Our chest begins to hurt. We try some antacid or maybe a glass of milk. We get worse. Fear starts to nag us. Maybe we are having a heart attack, maybe we are dying.

Do you see the drama that we have created? We failed to eat with consideration of the alkaline-acid balance of Nature for our dinner. We created our pain, our fear, and our reactions to that fear. But the drama is not over. There is now an intestinal track that is filled with acidic, fermenting waste. There is no fiber in that waste; there is only fat and other chemical waste. The fat the body can absorb, it does. The chemicals the body can absorb, so it does. The rest of the waste stays there getting dryer and harder.

Now we are in another drama – the drama of constipation. This, too, is a drama of our own creation. We have violated the Law of Nature that says our body must have oxygen, water, and plant material. We have violated the Law of Nature that says we need an 80 percent alkaline, 20 percent acid balance to the foods that we eat to provide the natural balance of the body to be maintained as the image of our health and happiness.

We are creating our own personal reality, but we may not recognize what we are doing. Creation requires drama, so let us look at this self who loves meat, potatoes, pie, and beer as a steady diet. We have the drama of indigestion, assimilation, and elimination. Our body has not received the foods of Nature that it needs to keep this alkaline-acid balance in the body, so we are functioning with a system that allows the organisms of our body to grow and flourish. One day we wake up with a cold. Our head aches, our nose is running, we are coughing, and our body aches all over. We are a miserable sight. We feel terrible again, but we have created a new drama. We are really sick! We have to stay in bed. We can't go to work. We are living our own personal creation.

These small dramas are the dramas of human life that we create and react to. They make our world what it is. This is possible primarily because we are unaware that we create a drama internally each time that we eat. As we can see, we set in motion a series of dramas that feed one into the other. As each tomorrow becomes today we repeat the drama. The physical insults can become a lifetime of physical abuse. Now we are 38 years old. We are overweight, have high blood pressure and only enough energy to be active during the hours that we have to work. We go to work, come home, eat a large meal – our favorite – sit down in our chair, watch television and go to sleep.

One night we awaken to move from our chair to our bed, and suddenly feel pain in our chest and arm. This time it seems worse than the average case of indigestion, but we swallow some pills and try to become comfortable. The drama rages on during the night, as we find ourselves in severe pain. We start to panic, knowing in our mind that we are facing death. Sure, we are afraid. Who wouldn't be? But the Doctors can fix it; all we have to do is get to the hospital before we die. Maybe this time they can help us. Maybe they can stretch the clogged blood vessels, or replace them. What we don't understand is they cannot heal us. They can keep us alive for a period of time with a lot of help from us, but we will live on drugs and we will continue to deteriorate.

We have learned to accept living in a state of disease. We have developed the belief system that disease is inevitable. We don't look at our health from the standpoint of understanding what we are doing wrong, or what creates the problem in the first place. We consider it part of our heritage as a human being. We have accepted no responsibility for our health. The mind that believes in disease creates disease. Identical dramas of fear, need and improper caring for the physical are the normal, everyday dramas of our world, especially in hospitals. They are created by the mental non-action and the physical reaction. The ingenuity of creation is endless within our continuing lives. Every human being needs to accept total responsibility for the food that we eat, the thoughts that we think and the dramas that we create. In more ways than one, we are creating our physical reality.

With the use of a simple steamer or patapar paper we can have a delicious meal that is nourishing for our body. Our diet should consist of at least six fruits a day and three of these should be citrus fruits. We also should have three green, yellow, or red vegetables that grow above the ground as well as one that is a tuberous vegetable for two meals. These can be taken hot at one meal and raw at another. Legumes, nuts and seeds are perfectly acceptable for our protein. Second generation foods should be limited in quantity as should third generation foods. They are not bad foods but they are further removed from Nature. These foods produce more waste material within the body and make it more difficult to maintain the proper balance of Nature. When they are used they should be consumed in the pure state and in addition to the vegetables and fruits.

Most people eat too much protein, fats, sugars and starches. This puts an increased burden on the natural balance and will create the daily dramas of dis-ease. Each and every cell within the body works from the concept of balance. If we eat all one food, we produce an excess of some elements and a deficiency of other elements. As the excess increases, the deficiency increases in Nature's system of balance. There is a significant mineral imbalance in our physical bodies today that is responsible for many of our physical problems. These problems are problems of mineral deficiency.

Our food processors are selling us foods that are destroying our physical body. The chemicals, preservatives, fats, sugars, and starches that are added to our foods are creating a serious imbalance in the physical self, which in turn creates an imbalance of mind and Spirit. Do not be hypnotized by words spoken purely for financial gain. Listen with discernment. It is our choice to accept and believe, or to not accept and not believe. Evaluate what you hear, see, and feel by the concept of the value to your life. If a product increases the value and happiness of your world, choose to use it. If it takes away from your world, either now or in the future, choose not to use it. Advertisements are not created for the benefit of our health and happiness. Advertisements are created to sell a product. The ability to evaluate rests with us. It is our choice. We can be well, or we can be sick and dying.

Drink fluids between meals not with meals. Diluting the hydrochloric acid in our stomach decreases the body's assimilation of nutrients. One glass of wine with a meal will aid in the digestion and assimilation processes. In this respect, red wine is more efficient than white wine. When taken in this manner it will help to build the body. Learn to spend your money on good natural foods, and you will find that you have a structural unit that is a functioning body unit. You will feel vital, alive, and full of beautiful health.

Our eating patterns have become so unbalanced with excesses, that the first step in changing the physical self is placing oneself on a cleansing dietary program. This does not require fasting, although for a sluggish body this is not detrimental for a twenty-four hour period. After that it becomes counter-productive, because the body needs to be restored, not starved. A person with a hyperactive body must never fast. It is damaging to the cellular structure. The ideal approach to this program is to follow it completely for a minimum of seven days. If you have excess weight or medical problems you can follow it for many weeks and it will be extremely beneficial despite current beliefs.

All infections are a problem of an imbalance in the alkaline-acid base within the body, which can be caused by excesses of some foods and deficiencies of others. In order to correct the alkaline-acid base of the body and to free the body of excessive waste material that has accumulated within the various systems of the body, the cleansing program of eating is essential.

It will not be detrimental to the body's physical health. It will provide the body with the organic mineral salts that it needs to restore cellular function. A change in the body's function can be noticed within the first week. This is true enlightenment for the body, when it realizes the mind has consciously accepted the responsibility of the physical self. As the mind builds, the physical body responds. Mealtime is a social custom and is not necessary for purposes of eating for cellular stability. We should eat when hungry from the foods of Nature. No other foods. We should eat less in quantity, chew slowly with peace, and eat small amounts more frequently, if our activity level is high.

Now that the commitment of the mind has been transferred into the action of the body, we are on the path to restoration of health. The cleansing program provides every element needed for the function of the body. It will not be seen in the proportions that our culture believes it to be needed, but our culture is one of the excesses. Changing from these excesses to the cleansing program will start us on our program of chemical balance.

The Cleansing Program

An Eating Process for the Joy of Health

AIR! AIR! AIR!

Practice deep abdominal breathing, in through the nose out through the nose, several times a day. This type of breathing allows the body to filter the air for you. Air is the force of life!

WATER! WATER! WATER!

Use fresh spring or well water without chemicals added. Drink a minimum of eight to twelve glasses per day. The human body is primarily water. Water is necessary for proper chemical balance.

FOODS OF NATURE!

Fruit! Minimum- Raw

2 grapefruits, 6 oranges, 3 lemons or limes (use as juice added to water)

Vegetables! Minimum

4 leafy green, red, yellow – Raw

4 leafy green, red, yellow – Steamed or Microwaved

Vegetables should be eaten in a ratio of 3-1, three grown above the ground to one grown in the ground. Eat all you can eat. We are not starving; we are cleansing and restoring the body. Do not eat: meats, breads, oils, butter, sugars, canned fruits, pastries, candies, eggs, milk, starches, legumes, potatoes, corn, grains, seeds and nuts during the cleansing program.

Eating is a process that is essential to maintenance of our physical body. If we fail to restore the organic mineral salts that are essential to the energy balance of the cells, our body will gradually cease to be. Our physical self is designed as a genius in cellular restoration. Our cells are replaced at least every seven years within every organ of our body. Many times we do not provide the proper material for the cells to work with. But in its programming, the body can convert many products into the exact needs of the body, if a portion of the proper elements is supplied. If the body does not receive these necessary elements, it will continue to convert to the best possible level from the elements it is given. Years of deficiency will add up to disease within the physical system.

A body that must function on a less than perfect level for years is destined for disease. The mind is building in an escape route. When living consciously with total awareness, we do not need an escape route. Our physical body will not be susceptible to viral, bacterial or other organism invasion, when it is in the proper alkaline-acid balance. Our body requires an 80 percent alkaline, 20 percent acid intake at its minimum, to withstand disease. During the diseased state, this ratio can be more efficient at a 90/10 ratio. This ratio gives the body the elements it has been deficient in, and uses the excesses for conversion material. The fruits and vegetables in Nature which are highly acid in character produce an alkaline reaction within the body. When we consume a variety of fruits and vegetables, we will be consuming those of varying degrees of alkalinity and acidity which will allow us to eat without worry. The proper balance will occur naturally.

Water and air are the most therapeutic elements in Nature. When they are added to the necessary plant foods, we will have the elements to change the cellular function of our body. Within time, our Earth will again recognize the therapeutic effects of fresh air, water and natural food. All disease can be cured with these elements, if our mind is willing. Water is an element that is also necessary for the body externally. It is the most calming of all therapies and could be used to much greater advantage in our medical world today.

During your period of the cleansing program, you have an activity program to begin. The first and foremost exercise of that program is total body movement. This can be done best with stretching exercises, swimming and walking. A bathtub and floor are available to most of you. Find a good set of stretching exercises that allows your body to move each and every muscle within. Do not overdo, but DO.

Before starting your daily exercise program either soak in a hot tub or take a hot shower. This will help you loosen up your muscles and prevent damage and soreness.

After your exercise, soak in comfortably hot water for thirty minutes. RELAX. If you have access to a swimming pool, don't forget to use it. Pools can be a problem because of too many chemicals, but it is better than nothing. Do not fear. If you have a swimming pool, use salt instead of chlorine, which will be healthier for you.

Walking is also a beneficial exercise, despite the fact that all muscles are not used. The primary advantage in walking is the breathing. This is the perfect time to practice deep breathing, and the closer you are to an uncontaminated environment the better for you. Being near water or open land is closer to Nature and closer to the real you.

With these activities controlled by a committed mind, you are well into your restoration regimen. Following a one to four-week period on the cleansing program, it is time for you to add more natural foods.

This program should become your LIFE PROGRAM. This is the proper way for us to eat, if we are interested in providing our body with the proper elements to insure maximum cellular function. This is the program where the mind builds the body and it must be maintained for life, if our final purpose is to truly understand the *Joy of Health.* The joy of health is the maximum balance of energy in body, mind and Spirit. Breathing fresh air, drinking pure water, and eating plant foods is supplying our bodies with Earth energy. Eating the wrong foods cheats our body of the vital elements that keep the body at its optimum state of function which is perfect physical health.

We are ENERGY. A light bulb is energy. When a light bulb transmits its energy, it glows. When the human body transmits its energy, it glows. There is no other way. Opening up the physical channels of energy allows the body, the mind and the Spirit to glow as one. For that ultimate glow of energy and health, begin to follow the Life Program of Natural Eating. The life program of natural eating requires that we continue to eat from the plants of the Earth. We can reduce the quantity from the cleansing program and add foods if we so desire. The secret of eating the natural way is in the preparation and choice of foods. Never focus your food intake on prepared foods, processed foods, and second or third generation foods. The focus should always be with the Earth's plants and their fruits and seeds. Protein can easily be obtained from these foods and as they are combined, the protein content increases. Oils should never be added to the diet but used only as they occur naturally within the foods. If we are creating a masterpiece that needs a little oil, use olive oil. An example of this is cold-pressed olive oil, which is good for the body when used in small amounts.

Processed foods have many oils added that cause destructive waste material to form within the body. Be conscious of these oils that produce many harmful effects within our physical system. At this period in our society, we do not understand or appreciate the damage we are inflicting within our physical self with the consumption of fats. Sugars and simple starches are also destructive to our health and should be consumed only as natural foods. The sugars of fruits and vegetables in their ripe state is a true natural food and beneficial. The sugar and starch of processed foods are destructive and responsible for many of our health problems. Examples of the sugar, starch influence are hypertension, diabetes, hyperactivity, indigestion, mental problems, high cholesterol, and stones. When the sugar, starch influence is combined with the fat influence, it becomes responsible for countless diseases directly and secondarily from the waste material produced that accumulates within the systems of the body.

The plant starches are found in beans, peas, corn, wheat, rice, barley, and more, which is in the seeds of the plant. In the early stages of these plants they are sprouts, which is a natural wealth of minerals. As the plant progresses they develop seeds and ripen, which produces protein and starch. Combining two of these foods together will give us a natural complete protein. The soybean can be used in place of milk, flour and meat. It should be a staple in our food intake. It is high in the minerals that we need for cellular balance. Our foods should never be genetically engineered by human beings. Genetic engineering changes their pure chemical balance.

Second generation foods should be used in their lean form, such as special cuts of beef, lamb and veal. Chicken, turkey and seafood have less fat and should be used more frequently. Second generation foods should be used at the maximum once daily in small quantities of one to three ounces. Large intakes of meat decrease the absorption of the plant minerals, as does the fat that the meat contains. The use of small quantities of meat for flavoring masterpieces from the soil is the best use of these second generation foods. But they can be used to accompany the vegetables of a meal, if the quantity is limited to the lean meats and consumed in small portions only once per day. Wild game is the meat of choice, if meat is used frequently. This, too, can interfere with assimilation, but the decrease in fat of the wild game partially decreases the interference. Wild game is also subjected to chemicals in relationship to their location.

Vegetables and fruits are true energy foods. This is not clearly understood by our world, but when Spirit put us in the Garden of Eden what were we given to eat? The apple tree was used as the symbol of the "Tree of Knowledge." The Garden of Eden was symbolic of our needs on the physical realm of Earth. Within that symbolism can be found the requirements of the physical, mental and Spiritual self. Today we feed our physical body from that symbolic "Tree of Knowledge." Also found in the Garden of Eden was the almond tree which was symbolic of the need for the minerals of the Earth.

The almond is one of Nature's most completely balanced foods and can contribute to the prevention of disease when used in the natural raw state.

The addition of third generation foods in the diet is more beneficial to all humans than the addition of second generation foods. We have viewed the egg as a problem. It is not the egg that raises our cholesterol, it is our other behaviors. The cholesterol or fat of Nature is better for us than the processed fats of our food industry. Processed fats combine with the starch and sugar in our foods to produce a low grade of cholesterol within the body. All fats should be used sparingly. Our body is programmed for Nature's elements. It is not programmed for the elements that we produce. The conversion process that is required on a cellular level can in this case produce an inferior element within the body. Inferior elements become waste material within our physical systems.

Third generation foods can be used in combination with first generation foods for nutritious and creative meals. Eggs add a true and easily digestible protein to the diet that is an advantage to health. A third generation food has integrated many of the elements of the Earth, because it is the reproductive seed for the second generation mother. We should not live on eggs alone, but we cannot live on any one food alone!

We can live a healthy physical existence on simply first generation foods. We can add third generation foods with some waste material being created, especially from the excessive use of cow's milk. Second generation foods will add waste material in even greater amounts unless used sparingly. When second generation foods and third generation foods are used in abundance, it is essential that first generation foods be used in even greater quantities to balance the needs of the physical self.

All foods above the third generation become foods produced by scientific knowledge and intellectual creativity. Avoid most of these foods. Food is not natural food, if it has been removed from its natural state of elemental mineral balance. Foods that have been added to, subtracted from, or changed from the character in which Nature presented them are processed food. The processed foods in our world are creating the state of physical imbalance or dis-ease that currently exists. Our processed foods are directly responsible for the high fat levels in our blood. These are foods of the mind. The mind is building a body from inferior material. Materials that do not conform to the Laws of Nature cannot be used to build the physical body in a state of total health.

First Generation Foods:

All foods grown from or within the Earth that are eaten in their natural state. These include all fruits, vegetables, seeds, grains, and nuts. This group also includes herbs that are used to enhance the flavor of foods and in some cases used as preventative or curative teas.

Second Generation Foods:

All animal, fowl, or fish that itself grows from eating the plants or other animals of Nature. These include beef, pork, lamb, veal, deer, rabbit, squirrel, turkey, chicken, quail, pheasant, dove, ducks, all fish, all seafood and others not necessarily mentioned.

Third Generation Foods:

All foods that are products of the reproductive systems of second generation foods. These include the eggs or seeds of second generation foods and the nectar they produce to feed their young. Nectars for the young are milk and honey.

Processed Foods:

Foods that are produced by man using a combination of first, second, and third generation foods that have been added to, subtracted from, preserved, dyed, and changed in character to produce a saleable product in the marketplace.

Life Program of Natural Eating:

Daily dietary intake: 80 percent totally natural first generation foods, 10 percent second generation foods in pure form, 10 percent third generation foods in pure form.

Season natural foods with fresh herbs, or the juice of lemon or lime. Do not use prepared seasonings, salt or sauces that are processed.

First generation foods can be creatively prepared with or without the use of second and third generation foods as condiments, if this is done within the home. These foods are then free of added fats, sugars, starches, chemicals, additives, preservatives or processing pollution and destruction. These foods will provide us with the most efficient digestion, assimilation and elimination through the needed elements of Nature. This pattern of natural eating will balance our body with the rhythm of Nature. Our energy flow will be in tune with the feeling-tones of the Earth. The mind and Spirit will open to the health of the physical, and the balance that we are searching for will be easy to reach. This is eating for restoration and balance.

Eat in good health!

Garden (Soul!) Salad

1½ c. whole grain brown rice
2 cans kidney beans
1 can fava beans
1 can chick peas
2 c. whole kernel corn
2 bunches parsley, finely chopped
1 pkg. green onions
2 garlic cloves, chopped fine
½ green pepper, chopped fine
½ red pepper, chopped fine
½ yellow pepper, chopped fine
Cilantro, finely chopped

Dressing

Juice from 4-6 lemons
1 T sea salt
½ c. olive oil

Substitute beans of choice, add vegetables of choice Broccoli, Tomatoes, Shredded carrots, Zucchini. Use plain chopped onions if green are not available.

DISEASES

This book is not written as a disease therapy manual but as an example of how our diseases are created. All diseases are created by the actions of how we process our foods and the actions of our mind, which result in the reaction of disease within our physical body. There is a well-defined coordination in the physical realm between the mind that builds the body, and the physical building blocks which we provide for our body in the food that we eat. All diseases known to us are the result of either excesses or deficiencies or a combination of both. These excesses and deficiencies occur in the lifestyle that we live, the thoughts that we create and the food that we eat. There are Laws of Balance and Compensation which function in coordination with the Law of Nature, on our physical plane of Earth. No one is exempt from these laws.

In our physical world someone who chooses to murder is subjected to the Law of Justice. This is a physical law that demands compensation and balance on a physical level for the murderer. In the Universal sense there are also Laws that require compensation and balance when they are not respected. If we murder our body with the insult of wrong eating, the Laws of Compensation and Balance will automatically go into operation. We will pay, just as the murderer will pay, for our actions.

Spirit has created upon Earth a cure for every disease that we can create. We cannot learn to heal ourselves until we create something to heal.

Healing must always be accepted by the mind before it will be created within the physical body. The cures that we see in our world today are cures first of the mind and secondly within the body. Medicine will effect a temporary relief from illness, because the mind belief is that medicine will cure. In reality medicine does not "cure," but it can provide temporary relief from symptoms. Only our mind can heal us. Healing requires a change in our belief system. A change in our belief system will create a change in our lifestyle.

Disease is a lesson for those who experience it. The creation of physical problems for ourselves during life is part of the lesson of physical existence. When we learn that disease is no longer essential to our lessons on Earth, disease will no longer be. Our lesson of physical existence is knowing that we can create our own reality with the actions or thoughts of the mind and the resulting reactions within the physical body. Our Spirit self allows us to experience the power of creation. We are our own creation from the moment of birth, just as each drama of our life is our own creation. The Soul purpose on Earth is always focused on learning these lessons for Soul evolution. The lessons themselves will differ from Soul to Soul, but the purpose of learning the lesson for Soul evolution will be the same for each. When this fact is understood on a Soul level, the lessons we learn will never need to be learned again. On Earth, true learning is unlearning. We must be willing to change our beliefs, if we want to grow.

Imagine Three Beautiful Castles

Understanding the bridge that exists between the mind and the body, and the concepts that are necessary to maintain this balance of Nature, will give us the physical longevity that will allow for consistent Soul evolution on Earth. There is a bridge between the mind and the body and the mind and the Spirit. Imagine three beautiful castles. They are several stories high and they each stand thirty feet apart but face each other in a circle. On every level of these three castles, there is a bridge that is built of the same sturdy construction of stone and mortar which reaches out from each castle to become a part of the other castles. Each castle is separate but they are one. They appear as one and they function as one. In the physical world we can view them as one beautiful castle. The bridges that connect these three separate castles are equivalent to the bridges of consciousness that connect our body, mind and Spirit. The primary bridge in this connection, for all of us, is our Dual Soul.

The castle is integrated into one functioning unit. If the lights go out in one part of the castle they go out everywhere. To function properly the body must be recognized as an integrated unit of three distinct parts.

We cannot function well if we isolate ourselves in one room of the "castle." If we accept our self as only the physical body, the other two wings of the castle are going to fall into dis-repair and the entire castle will be compromised. The castle may disintegrate if repair work is not done equally and immediately to pull the castle together again into an integrated unit. When we focus only on one part of the self, or two parts of the self, the remaining part of the self is falling into disrepair. It has entered the danger zone and it will bring the rest of us to the ground as it tumbles.

It is within that physical structure of the castle that the physical power exists. The physical integration controls the heat, the electricity, the building power of the three castles. The physical castle creates a structure for the function within the interior of the castles. If we focus on the physical self and the mental self and ignore the Spiritual self, we will create a disaster within our physical castle. If we focus on the mental and the Spiritual self and ignore the physical, we will create a disaster within our physical castle. If we focus on the physical and Spiritual self without the mental input, we will create disaster to our physical castle. This is the Law of Cause and Effect. We, as human beings, cause the "happenings" within self. Disease is the effect of being out of balance. All effects will eventually be manifested within the physical, because we are living within the physical realm. We cannot avoid this effect.

Looking at our world from the physical level will reveal our concept of eating behaviors that allow us to produce disease within our body. These are the immediate reactions to our thoughts and beliefs that create our physical self. Have you ever heard anyone say, "I am an emotional eater"? This is a conscious admission that the mind is controlling the body. Most eating and not eating is an emotional reaction. We have lunch with someone and we eat because of the emotion of sharing the experience, not because we are hungry. Many times we use eating as a reason to share time with friends. It is part of our belief system, and it is pleasant and happy for us. Do not stop doing something that is a happy experience. The example is being given only to trigger our awareness.

Any person who chooses not to eat is also reacting to an emotion. This can be the emotion of unworthiness in the same way that eating can be from the emotion of unworthiness. The emotions are identical in nearly every case. The reaction to the emotion is individualized. The body is the physical product that shows the direct influence of one unit upon another unit. As we compromise the energy output of one unit it acts to affect the energy output in the other units. We consistently receive a result for each action. The reaction to the denial of Spirit is addiction to alcohol, drugs, eating, sex, smoking, lying, cheating, and criminal behaviors.

We will attempt to balance this need for Spirit with a substance that is within the physical realm. The Spiritual self is out of balance. Addiction is a mental reaction and a physical response. There is no Spiritual involvement in addiction; therefore, there is denial and resistance to the Spirit self. This is an easy imbalance to recognize. An awareness of what we are doing and an understanding of why we are choosing this action will start us on the path to balance and health. Looking internally for the core cause of disease requires truth and love of self.

Fear, anger, hate and guilt are all mind actions that allow us to punish ourselves with disease. In the Spiritual sense, anger, hate and guilt are all reactions to fear. Fear is a negative energy force. It is the opposite of love. Therefore, if we exist in fear we do not have that love of self and our fellow human that is Spirit's basic message.

The basis of all fear is the fear of separation from Spirit. This is our subconscious Soul reminding us that we do not love ourselves as Spirit, and our neighbor in the same like manner. Facing oneself and the fear within in a straight-forward manner will allow us to find the sense of love that we deserve and essentially have, but are failing at the moment to acknowledge. Our belief system has taught us to fear. We fear separation: the separation of a spouse, a job, a friend, a child, a lover, and the list can go on and on in our world. This same fear can motivate us to have a disease which can work to avoid separation, to bring us love and attention and to protect us at all costs. Of course this will not protect us. It is only an illusion of protection within our mind. The other people in our world will not be affected by us in the same way that our body is being affected. They will tolerate our constant complaints, sometimes gracefully, sometimes not so gracefully, but the effect of our dis-ease will impact us and everyone that is around us.

An illusion is a false belief that we are attached to. The way to change our actions is to change our belief, our illusion. This will be our healing energy. Disease can also be freely chosen as a lesson with no fear in the process of disease, death or dying. When disease is chosen simply as a lesson of patience, for example, an inner peace exists within us. There is no fear, no anger, no guilt, and no sadness. There is only acceptance and the need to learn and be while in the process of the disease and dying. The disease itself is not the lesson. The lesson is learning patience. A Soul that has chosen disease for any personal lesson not based in fear will never be found in self-pity or anger.

Learning the lesson of healing is another reason to choose disease. This is working directly with the coordination of the body and mind. We cannot learn to heal ourselves until we create something to heal. We create and heal many diseases without medical intervention. When this happens this Soul has already accepted the responsibility for self. Accepting responsibility is not his lesson. Healing self is his lesson.

Another type of fear of separation is the fear of separation of self. This is also seen as a basis of fear because self is the Spirit self. This fear is manifested when a Soul sees himself as being controlled, suppressed, or defenseless with another person. This person will create a disease that will suppress the function of self. The diseases are many times chronic diseases such as arthritis, a multitude of muscle and nerve diseases, and asthma. Many of these diseases will be accompanied by alcoholism which will worsen the disease.

Separation from self is a true separation from Spirit, the Spirit self that may not be acknowledged and therefore may go unrecognized in the list of fears. The only cure for all disease is a Spiritual awakening that will allow us to totally change our belief system and our lifestyle. Anytime there is the fear of separation from Spirit, there is an extreme resistance to understanding and change that is created by the ego self. This resistance and denial keeps us from understanding that we are responsible for our own creation of self.

This fear is felt many times when we find ourselves in a position that we find unacceptable to our internal value system of honesty, truth and productivity. We will become subconsciously aware, often gradually, that we cannot be in that environment and function as we are supposed to function without the need to compromise our own sense of eternal ethical values. This fear will generate many reactions on a physical level. We may become seriously ill, we may gain weight, we may decide to drink more than we should, or some other manifestation will appear. We may never become aware of the situation we are creating for ourselves physically by remaining in the situation. We may lose our job because of drinking too much, because of our chronic illness, because we didn't come to work many days out of the month. Through all of the problems that exist, we will resist change. The subconscious Soul is screaming for acknowledgement, and the ego is resisting change.

The mind will try to create a situation to protect our body and Spirit. The intuitive part of our mind is aware of the circumstance. It sees the Soul and the ego at total war within. The situation will be created, whether or not it is understood on a physical level. The entire battle of self is being recorded in the physical body and will manifest itself as a form of disease. Our mind is ingenious in its fear. Addictions are a common way of dealing with fear. Addiction is a suppression of self. Addiction is imprisonment of our Soul and Spirit. We search for freedom while creating imprisonment. Most of us are willing to destroy our physical self, rather than deal with the internal agony of the fear of separation from Spirit. The way of destruction is determined by our ego. The way is unimportant, it is only a path. Destruction is the end result of all disease or addiction. Destruction is the goal. Why would we want to destroy ourselves? Because we feel unworthy in the eyes of Spirit. Understanding that we are perfect just as we are at the Spirit level of self is necessary for us to heal ourselves. *Learning to love ourselves for our true self is the first step in the transition from fear to love and from disease to health.* Health is the path to vibrant well-being. Health is the opposite of disease. All of life experience is a lesson in opposites. As human beings, we cannot miss any lesson that our Dual Soul is determined that we must learn and live.

Acts of Love

Feeding our body the natural foods that will give us strength and energy is an act of love to self. Eating for health is the perfect place to start in our physical focus. The benefits of this are twofold, because the increased energy and sense of well-being gives us a better self-image and makes it easier to continue the love of self, which is always our healing energy. With this healing energy we can cure all diseases.

This can be the beginning of our disease-free, vibrant health cycle. We deserve it. We are perfect in every respect. If we are a substance addict, restoration of the physical self is essential to freeing the physical body from the imprisonment of the substance. Fear and poor nutrition are so tightly intermingled in the disease process that we cannot talk about them individually. All of our diseases are the result of the imbalance of the mind, body and Spirit of self. This imbalance causes the excesses and deficiencies to occur. The excesses and deficiencies of eating, drinking and lifestyle impact the physical body and therefore they impact our health. When we eat foods that no longer contain the elements that our body needs, we begin a disease cycle that can result in a death cycle. Change is always the common denominator that has the wisdom to heal our human body.

If we believe that our diseases are caused by germs, we are only partially correct. The lower organisms that exist in our world were created when we were created. We normally live in harmony with the lower organisms of the Earth and our body. When the balance within us is lost, the lower organisms become virulent to us. We have created a phenomenon known in Nature as the survival of the fittest. Organisms will grow naturally in a body that has the correct balance. The stomach itself is highly germicidal and naturally kills ingested organisms, if the body is truly in balance. The correct alkaline-acid balance of each and every cell of the physical body is necessary to true health. There are millions of organisms in our Universe and we live with them compatibly, unless we lower our physical body's resistance and give them the atmosphere they need to flourish. Our resistance is lowered by our mind, and our body responds. This is why the medical community should study healthy people or people who quickly overcome disease, rather than the diseases or diseased people themselves. We already understand that we have disease.

We must study our miracles of healing! Change is the true miracle of life and healing.

Research on any group of people who have experienced what we would call miracle healings would show that the first thing they did was to start eating naturally, changed their lifestyle and their attitude toward their life and living. They began to feel differently about themselves internally, and they began to relate differently to the rest of their world. They began to love themselves and their neighbor. They began the process of balancing the body, mind and Spirit of self. They made a conscious decision to be healthy. They chose life. The lesson the Dual Soul learned from the disease was an individual lesson. The lesson itself may have been different for each person who has ever undergone a healing. The difference in the lessons is unimportant. The understanding of healing is the important lesson that is Universal. Learning the lesson so that it never returns as a lesson is the goal of healing. All humans have the power to heal diseases in their body, which is balancing their thinking, emotions, and senses to support their internal growth.

What is a miracle healing? In your world this is defined as a healing that cannot be scientifically explained. Study the people who have experienced miracle healings and they can be explained. No healing will ever occur without change. This change may not be in the form of scientific therapy or medicine, as we define it, but if we truly communicate with the healed, we will hear about the changes of the thinking mind, which is reflected into the body and Spirit. The change is always found within our belief system. Change is the true miracle of healing.

If you find yourself in a situation where you want to heal yourself, it is important to know that "Change is the miracle of healing." When we are ill we must look at our level of happiness and our behaviors. Where are we being challenged? Are we challenged at work, in our personal life, in our profession or in any aspect of our existence? Look at your world carefully. Disease usually says that "You are living in fear." Search for the problem and change it. What is the belief attachment that is holding us captured within the energy of fear? Remember that the root cause of fear is the fear of separation from Spirit. Who do we identify as our Spirit?

Fear is the beginning and the end of us as energy in physical terms. Until we acknowledge that something is wrong and change it, whether or not we totally understand the "something," the effect upon our body will be there. Find the cause and we can remove the effect, if we are willing to change. It is always important to remember that our life is about learning. If we deny learning in this life, we will create the same problem in our next life, but we will increase our fears to capture our attention.

Health professionals are today's healers. They have chosen to care about people. They are here to teach others to care, as well as to guide in the understanding of healing. Their teachings may temporarily be stuck in the mechanistic, materialistic concept that they have been taught, but on a Soul level they are capable of sensitivity and creativity towards all human beings. We are energy beings, and when we can balance our energy, we can heal ourselves. The true need to be a physician is a Soul need to learn the fine art of healing ourselves. Our society generates educational choice usually by emphasizing financial rewards and status, but for the true physician money and fame are not the motivation.

Nurses are entirely motivated by the caring they feel for others. They are open-minded Souls with clear paths of evolution. In our society there is more financial motivation now than ever before for those who have chosen nursing. They are the caretakers in the health care community. For them the path has been challenging and joyful. Many have chosen the happiness of caring for others over marriages, money, fame and glory. Our present societal concept of medicine has such a strong hold on our medical world, that physicians, nurses and other health care professionals find themselves pressured by people demanding instant cures. This is not a reality from within the mind of the person who accepts responsibility for self. All true healing is from within. Death gives us an opportunity to begin a new life with rebirth.

There are young and unaware Souls who feel that the responsibility for their creation is with another, rather than themselves. They have many lessons to learn. Anger and blame are their response to their own guilt and fear. We create guilt and anger because we feel negligent and unworthy in caring properly for ourselves or our loved one. We must find another to blame for our unworthiness, because we have not learned to accept the responsibility for our own actions. It is our lesson.

There are many new Souls on Earth at this time. The new Soul has not reached the awareness of love. The new Soul operates on the Earth level, primarily out of fear. This fear is the ultimate fear of separation from the physical body. We are taught to be terrified of death. On a subconscious level we know there is much to be learned. But we have not accepted the eternity of our Spirit on a conscious level. We do not know that there is no death, there is only living. Living has no opposite. Living was created by Spirit, and what Spirit has created cannot be changed. Death is a physical illusion. Death is in reality the freedom to choose again by creating a new body and continuing with life. This young Soul believes that he has only one change. He is out there struggling against the world to make certain that he gets his due. Souls may have had many, many Earth incarnations, but until they begin to develop through the understanding of experience, they remain unevolved Souls that cannot in any way understand themselves. These Souls are essentially new Souls in the concept of development not in the concept of creation.

A morbid fear of death will bring death to the physical body. The mind will build the body with that response being created. Guilt, fear, anger, hate and all other negative emotions will have the same physical response. This mind concept will be created within the physical self. We will make it come true. While the mind is creating the physical, it will also be creating the Spiritual. Emotions of fear send out negative energy into our aura or energy field that surrounds our body and increases disease. This negative energy will attract negative energy. At the same time that we may be experiencing physical disease, we will be attracting other negative forces into our life, which might keep us from healing ourselves.

An example of this would be finding yourself physically ill, without money, having a car that breaks down, or alone as your spouse leaves you. If this has happened to you, it is time for introspective Soul searching and love. We alone have the ultimate power of creation for ourselves, and we can change anything that happens in our reality. This does not include making other people conform to our needs. It applies only to self. We have the choice of change. We are responsible for the creation. There are two diseases in our world today that are both the direct and extreme result of fear. These two diseases are cancer and AIDS. Extreme fear requires extreme diligence in proper nutrition, to maintain the proper alkaline-acid balance which is totally out of balance in these diseases. Both diseases are curable, but it requires a complete change in attitude and understanding as well as a total revision of lifestyle and eating habits.

AIDS:

In AIDS the fear is manifested in guilt, but the true fear is the fear of separation from Spirit which is secondary to the belief in punishment for the guilt that might be felt. Spirit does not sit in judgment of how one chooses to learn his lessons. Homosexuality is an extreme example of a true "identity crisis." Homosexuality is the ultimate in confusion regarding the identity of self. All humans are ultimately searching for their eternal personal Dual Soul identity and how to relate to other people. Our true human identity is the Spirit self. Acknowledgement of the Spirit self provides the balance, the understanding of self that we are seeking. As a Dual Soul our true fear is our "separation from Spirit." When anyone chooses to live in a manner that has been thought to be wrong by his belief system, he will be overcome by guilt and the fear of punishment, which is reflecting his Dual Soul lessons.

It doesn't matter how many people who read this say, "I have no guilt, or fear." Believe me when I say that deep down within the mind, Spirit and Soul of you, you most certainly do. You are a Human. You are the product of a belief system. This belief system has been supported by our "religions" since the beginning of our world. We believe in punishment for guilt and sin, even when we deny that belief. Our actions of homosexuality are an open denial to the world that we deny Spirit and the power of Spirit. Homosexuality is a form of sexual addiction. All addictions are caused by a fear of the separation from Spirit. We may consciously feel that we no longer subscribe to those beliefs, but we have not learned the lesson of freedom from beliefs or of self-love, because if we had we would not have created the illness of sexual addiction. We would no longer be searching for our identity. Anyone who is secure in his identity is secure within. There is no search within or without. All forms of sexual addiction are equivalent to any other disease of the human mind and Spirit. They are created by an imbalance within the body, mind and Spirit of self. They are our creation for the lessons of all human beings.

The Spirit self is a balanced self. It is male, it is female. It is total integration of body, mind and Spirit. As humans we naturally seek our mate in the opposite sex because it creates physical balance. We are each male and female, as manifested by the Dual Soul mind as the symbolic male and the Spirit as the symbolic female. We cannot be separated; we are one as a male and female energy. The physical identity for any one incarnation is chosen as to sex before the Soul enters Earth. We are always, as Dual male and female Souls, seeking balance. When we choose other than that which balances us, we are simply and clearly working on the lesson of balance in this incarnation.

The disease of AIDS is created by imbalance. It is created by the imbalance in the mind and spirit, which impacts on the imbalance created within the body and mind by the sexual relationship. When it is accepted as the true lesson that it is, the belief system can be changed and the sexual addiction will be healed. The physical body can then be balanced through the proper thinking and nutrition, so the organism that is ravaging the body will cease to live in that body. The physical self will not survive without the understanding of the lesson. *The only true cure for addiction is a Spiritual awakening. There is no other way.*

The Soul that chooses homosexuality is a Soul that is avoiding the issue of balance of the Spirit self. It is a Soul that is confused in the male, female balance within. The fear that this Soul externalizes is the fear of inadequacy or unworthiness on a physical level. Fearing inadequacy or sexual unworthiness in the role of the male makes avoidance of that balance an easier choice on the Earth plane. Homosexuality is a choice. Because homosexuality is a choice, it does not impact within our legal system. Other sexual addictions do impact within the legal system of our world, because they do not involve choice of both parties, especially where children are concerned.

The creation of AIDS is also the choice of the homosexual, because it is the next step in trying to understand the creation of balance within the physical body. Those who have chosen AIDS have chosen it as a way to abort a life that is not working to create that balance for the Soul. There is excitement in danger. The danger of AIDS and the reality of AIDS were created by the male homosexual energy within the Universe in an attempt to force the lesson of physical and chemical balance. All lessons require a change within the belief system, and a balancing of the body, mind and Spirit of self. This also holds true in the female role of homosexuality. Avoidance is an Earth manifestation of fear. Inadequacy is a fear by illusion. How can you be inadequate in a relationship where there is already male and female within each participant? On the physical level we are first seeking a balance of the physical, which will allow us to create a balance of the mind and Spirit. There is nothing to fear more than the fear itself. Inadequacy and unworthiness are both illusions of our mind that are related to our beliefs. Anytime that we feel we are living in a state of imbalance, we are conscious of how our "energy" feels in a state of imbalance, which makes us feel that change is essential. Becoming balanced in our energy is our challenge.

The concepts of unworthiness and inadequacy are products of our society's belief systems. The illusion of not being able to live up to the ideals of society's dictates is a manifestation of a poor self-image. It is believing in the illusion of conformity as a necessary part of living. It is not understanding and loving the human self, as the creator that is within us. It is not accepting our own balance. It is not understanding that we should not try to live by anyone's belief system except the one that is within us as our Spirit self. Inadequacy and unworthiness are both judgment calls of the individual based upon our belief system. Finding balance in life is finding someone who has the same balance, where the energy balance that is ours is in rhythm with the energy balance of the other person. This does not create inadequacy or unworthiness, it creates joy and happiness between two balanced Souls. This is balancing the mind. Heterosexuality is balancing the body. Homosexuality is incapable of balancing our physical self; therefore, the balance this Soul may feel in the mind becomes an illusion of balance which is frequently the energy bleed-through from a past life. This precarious balance will be subjected to extremes in emotional upheaval. Each Soul has many lessons to learn in each incarnation. They are lessons and the way they are learned is not to be judged, because the lesson must be lived. There is no wrong. There is only choice and the experience of life.

The nutritional program that will restore the body in all diseases is the same program that is given in this book for cleansing the body of disease and waste matter. After this program has been completed, the Soul needs to eat a balanced intake as outlined in the maintenance eating program. This program is Nature's creation to restore and revitalize the physical body and mind. It will not be effective in those Souls who fail to make the mental adjustment that is essential to health. Despite this limitation, it can provide a healthy way of eating for every human being.

Cancer

Cancer, too, is a disease of fear. The root of the fear is different in different people, but for many it is an inability to love self. There is a fear of rejection and inadequacy that may descend into the mind of a Soul that truly does not have self-love. Cancer can be used as an escape from the present life, when the lack of self-love instills that feeling of hopelessness into the Soul mind and emotions.

Cancer is also a disease that is chosen by many Souls as a lesson of the physical. Lessons of the physical are the lessons of the attributes of joy in the physical world. Some examples are patience, trust, faith, understanding, caring, sharing and others of equal importance, which they have chosen to learn under the stress of disease. For instance, a Soul who is an extreme introvert, who cannot accept love, sharing, caring or show patience towards his fellow man, who does not meet the belief standards that he judges them on, may decide to learn all of these lessons by putting herself/himself in the position of being very ill with cancer. In this position he is forced to accept caring, patience, love, non-judgment and sharing from the rest of the world. This Soul is placing himself in a position of need, to learn from others. There are other ways to learn these lessons. But a Soul who has incarnated many times, with the same basic list of lessons to learn without learning them, may make the choice to go all the way and learn from disease.

Lessons that become chronic or repeated in the life design at the time of birth are known in our world as Karma. A Soul can decide to erase Karma, at any cost, during an incarnation. If we don't succeed in other ways, we may choose cancer as our final choice of learning and growing. The world will see a Soul on the surface that is different from the internal self-image of the Soul. The true self-image, as manifested within the ego, will be one of hopelessness and despair. One physical manifestation that will be apparent is periods of depression. A Soul that lives in joy will not usually choose cancer as a lesson. If they do, it will not be a lingering illness for that Soul.

Deeply rooted self-image problems create eating problems that feed into the development of cancer as a disease. Souls with self-image problems will eat large amounts of red meat. They will crave the strength of the meat to create strength within them. They will also crave sugar in some form, either sweets or alcohol, to act as immediate energy. They envision their energy source from the external rather than the internal. Their self-image does not allow the utilization of the internal energy of the Spirit Consciousness. Their diet does not provide and indeed robs them of the minerals and nutrients of Nature, which are essential to viable cellular function. Large amounts of protein interfere with the absorption of nutrients and minerals within the body. Protein contains no fiber and it satisfies the appetite, decreasing the consumption of other natural foods. These individuals do not eat the bulk roughage to eliminate properly and frequently suffer from constipation. Poor elimination allows reabsorption of the poisons from their diet to become toxins within their system. Any waste matter from the diet that is not digested, assimilated and eliminated according to the needs of Nature can be the physical core cause of disease. Eating habits create our excesses as well as our deficiencies in nutrition.

Large amounts of protein interfere with the absorption of Nature's electromagnetic energy in foods. Sugar that is not within Nature's food itself interferes with the absorption of nutrients. Large amounts of alcohol, carbonated beverages, and food preservatives will deplete the nutrients and minerals from the body. Digestion, assimilation and elimination are keys to our physical health and the prevention of our chronic diseases. Digestion begins in the mouth as a physical process. Saliva is highly alkaline in nature and is the first step in the digestive process. The thorough chewing of food provides the mechanical dissolution mixed with the alkaline saliva that begins the process of the alkaline-acid balance. Those who claim to eat right but still have indigestion do not chew thoroughly. They have missed their first step in the alkalization process.

Digestion will be interfered with if liquids are taken with a meal, other than a small glass of wine. The grape sugar of a good wine is indeed a food and enhances digestion and assimilation unless it is used excessively. Other liquids should be used one hour before and one hour after a meal. Drinking water, tea or coffee at meal time dilutes the hydrochloric acid in our stomach which interferes with the digestive process. Some people will tolerate this dilution better than others, depending on the foods being consumed and the chewing that takes place.

Assimilation is a sensitive process, as we have discussed, and can be placed in a tremendous state of imbalance by many chemicals, drugs, and processed foods. Processed foods have most of Nature's nutrients removed, but the few remaining nutrients may not be absorbed because of the preservatives, chemicals, fats, and sugars that have been added to the food. Improper intake, poor assimilation and poor digestion are the beginnings of our disease process.

Poor elimination is the next promoter of disease. By nature we should eliminate three to four times a day depending upon the amount of food that was ingested. These should be stools of bulk that move smoothly through the intestinal tract. Elimination is the removal of waste material from the intestinal tract. If you eat large amounts of food, you should have large amounts of waste. The concept of daily or weekly elimination is a concept of improper eating habits and disease. It is a promoter of early physical problems and disease in later life. Many cancers are secondary to poor elimination, where the body harbors the waste material too long, which releases the toxins from the waste material into the blood stream. The person that eats of Nature's foods and drinks the water the body needs will find himself with more frequent eliminations and less physical disease.

Constipation, which is a true promoter of cancer, is our world's most chronic health problem. It promotes the use of more drugs than any other physical problem in our society. These drugs in turn compound the problem of digestion and assimilation. Constipation must be recognized as a symptom of improper eating habits and drinking habits. Anyone that is constipated should make certain that they routinely drink eight full ten ounce glasses of water a day and more if it is indicated to create daily elimination. In itself, constipation is not a disease. It is a created condition. Proper eating of raw fruits and vegetables will usually prevent both constipation and diarrhea. Diarrhea, too, is a created condition. It is caused by improper intake, poor digestion and poor assimilation. The cause is the same, although the body reacts differently in different individuals. Each of these symptoms is created daily by the individual.

Cancer is the combined problem of fear, poor eating habits, digestion, assimilation, and elimination. The root of these problems exists in the mind and their reactions are within the body, especially in the intestinal system. Souls with a poor self-image many times look upon elimination with guilt. They literally hold their waste material in for strength, and feel guilt at allowing it to leave their bodies. This is a fearful Soul that is hiding self and all creations of self. We can only solve this nagging problem by learning everything that we can possibly learn about ourselves and our journey in life, which will release our fear of both life and death. Normally these individuals will believe intensely that we live only one physical life, and they will have a morbid fear of death.

They also hold their emotions in and feel that communication and sharing will allow others to know who they really are. They live with the concept that they will not be loved if people really know them as they know themselves. They feel, on a conscious level, their unworthiness, inadequacy, and guilt. This is the guilt of the mind. Everything is held tightly inside, so the world cannot see. These Souls will gravitate to a diet of little bulk and little water. They will make laxatives a part of their daily life. These laxatives increase poor assimilation and poor digestion. This can be seen dramatically demonstrated with our older population. Fear is an emotion that freezes us into a form of stasis, keeping the organs in our body from functioning properly, which creates many diseases.

This can also be observed as an opposite reaction, where the bowels will stay in an uproar, because the emotions are in an uproar internally. This situation also creates problems with digestion, assimilation and elimination. We are searching for balance in life as well as in bodily functions. The bodily function is the physical manifestation of the mind. In diarrhea or diseases of colitis, our fear is creating the excesses or diseases of colitis, and our fear is creating the excesses of elimination. Any form of diarrhea requires a high bulk diet to normalize the constant spasm of the intestines, and to allow the body to function normally as it is designed to function.

All human Souls with cancer need to open their body, mind, and Spirit to the joy of life. They need to share their fears and search to understand and love themselves. They need to join support groups to realize they are not alone in their fears and in their feelings. Their fear of rejection and their poor self-image needs the reinforcement of sharing and caring from other Souls. They need support in learning to eat the proper foods to restore their cellular function with the proper alkaline-acid balance. They need support in seeing the world differently, and enjoying it with a freedom and openness they have never known before. Their fear is holding them prisoner, internally and externally.

The healing energy of understanding and support will start the internal process of the mind and Spirit flowing together. The change in nutrition will change the physical process, as the body finds a new balance with the foods of Nature. The cleansing program of eating will begin the physical cleansing to rid the body of the cancerous waste material. Progressing to the second generation foods will add variety to the daily intake to provide the strength and joy we all need to enjoy and expand our physical lives.

Psoriasis & Arthritis

Two other diseases that we will cover are Psoriasis and Arthritis, which seem to be basically incurable in our world. They cause many people overwhelming mental and physical agony.

All diseases are a lesson for the Dual Soul, and the lesson is universally individual. These chronic diseases cause tremendous pain both physically and mentally, but the lessons that are learned in the experience of disease are overwhelmingly positive. Lessons are never singular in manifestation because the body and mind work in coordination. We are one, we cannot be separated. Because of this there is always coordination between the mind and Spirit, even when it is resisted and denied. When we have any form of disease we must look very carefully at our physical life to see the lesson that we are learning.

People with multiple diseases are Souls who should and must stay close to Mother Earth to balance themselves chemically. Psoriasis and Arthritis are both diseases of the connective tissue which holds the body together, symbolic of our body, mind and Spirit which holds us together. These individuals need to restore their bodies from the Earth and enjoy the virtues of the soil, sun, and sea. This is beneficial to all bodies, but to these Souls it is crucial to health.

Here are three extremely important points for the Soul to remember in caring for the physical self:

Drink at least 64 ounces of water each day.

Remove all processed food from the diet.

Eat large amounts of raw foods high in ascorbic acid.

The raw foods of Nature will provide the electromagnetic energy to restore the body's connective tissue. The acids found in processed foods and drinks, coffee, tea and alcohol will not be good for these physical bodies.

For many Souls that have chosen these diseases, the lesson is one of patience and non-judgment. These are two lessons of higher Soul evolution, which we all must learn. They are each lessons of a lifetime, and for many they are lessons of many, many incarnations. The lessons do come back as Karma for many Souls. To create them as a twin lesson within one incarnation is in itself a lesson in patience.

Psoriasis

Souls who have chosen Psoriasis to help them learn must stay closely attuned to the Earth, eating large amounts of green leafy vegetables and fresh fruits, especially citrus fruits. Protein should be limited to four ounces daily and should be eaten frequently in the form of fish. The nutrients we know as Vitamin A and Vitamin C are needed in large quantities, but they must be obtained from the foods of the soil and the sea. Chemical preparations are never good for these Souls. The alkaline-acid balance of the body will be the one thing that will allow for clearness of the skin and control of the problem. All natural acids from the fruits of the Earth are highly alkaline within the body and should be used in abundance. Chewing foods thoroughly is essential as the first step in alkalizing the body. The vegetables of the Earth contain large amounts of organic mineral salts that are essential to the health of the skin.

Processed foods should be avoided, as they contain chemicals, preservatives, fats, sugars and starches that will change the body to an acid balance. For people with psoriasis, processed food is a cross to bear in life. We have many and various reactions to the dyes, chemicals, preservatives, and rancid fats that are found in processed foods. Living from these foods is an invitation to disease. Many diseases and deaths are related to these foods but they go unrecognized or unacknowledged by our society. We have removed ourselves too far from the rhythm of Nature. But as we age, our body will be challenged to maintain health at the level that it chooses, unless we can understand these issues and live accordingly. Fats, sugars and starches are highly acid foods within the physical body. The only fats that should be used are the natural fats within the foods of the Earth. Fats that are processed, with the exception of cold-pressed olive oil, should be avoided.

We should eat Jerusalem artichokes several times a week, and it is best if grown from the land on which we live. The acid that is found in coffee and tea is harmful to the body and should be avoided. Coffee that is made fresh from the coffee bean is acceptable in small quantities when the skin is clear. Processed coffee is never acceptable, as the acid content is too high. Pesticides sprayed on coffee beans add to the acid and other cumulative toxins in our system.

Pure water is essential in the lives of each and every Soul, but for this Soul it is the elixir of the Spirits. It should be consumed frequently throughout the day in its purest form. It should be enjoyed for soaking, showering and swimming, as well as drinking. Water can wash our troubles away as we ingest it and use it for pleasure and exercise such as swimming. Once the Soul is free of symptoms he/she can enjoy an occasional indiscretion without worry, but it must not become a habit. Variety will avoid depletion of the electromagnetic energy forces that are crucial to the health of this Soul.

These Souls are searching Souls and need to give themselves the opportunity to grow and search. They must spend quiet time with Nature, digging in the dirt, walking on the beach, swimming, hiking, lying in the sun. They need to meditate and luxuriate. They need peace. It is wise to be in peaceful surroundings during work and play. Stress will cause unbalance within the mind and body of these Souls. Many have a tendency to focus their energy on other people which is their caring nature. But in their caring, they must not forget to care about the Self. Happiness, joy and self-appreciation will make it easier for the body to rejuvenate. Reduce all external and internal stress. Take time for daily introspection. You deserve it. Give it to you as a gift to yourself.

Arthritis

Arthritis can show a miraculous physical change with a change in the nutritional intake and the exercise level. This will be more complete and permanent if the Soul searches for self-understanding. The Soul that has chosen Arthritis has chosen physical suppression. This Soul fears moving forward in life. It fears change. The physical pain is the resistance to moving forward. Arthritis is a physical disease of both excesses and deficiencies that is manifested by a reaction to both waste material in the body and a compromised cellular function.

In the mind, Arthritis is a disease of oppression. This Soul has lost sight of its eternal sense of freedom and has allowed itself to believe that freedom no longer exists. When you lose the freedom of the Spirit and the thinking mind, it will always be manifested in the loss of freedom of the body. This loss that starts as a feeling of oppression grows into a fear of failure. The Soul then is afraid of freedom. Movement is freedom. Trying is freedom. Changing is freedom. Going forward is freedom.

The mind control can occur at any point in the incarnation of the Soul. When it occurs in infancy, it is the freedom of the Spirit that is being oppressed. That Soul is struggling with the oppression of the physical body. The Soul is not comfortable with the physical body. There is a question in the child of returning to the Spirit world. As the child lives, it will be consciously making its choice to either stay or leave.

Arthritis may appear to a young mother with children. Her freedom is restricted to her on a physical, mental, and perhaps Spiritual level, as she is restricted to the task of raising children. Restriction is always an illusion of the mind. The freedom of the Spirit and Soul is never restricted. In the case of this young mother there can be a restriction of the physical and mental if she allows it to be. Her challenge is in the coordination of the mind and Spirit. This will allow her the freedom within her physical self.

Arthritis may occur in the business man who finds himself restricted to the task of making money, when he truly wants to go walk on the beach and dream. He has set his priorities in life, and his belief in those priorities restricts him. If he changes his belief, he changes his restriction, and his arthritis can be healed. Change is always forward movement, even if that is not accepted by our society's belief system. Without change we can only live in stasis. Our stasis of thought is our most damaging Dual Soul injury, therefore we must be conscious of our growth and change to avoid this form of stasis.

Arthritis may occur in later life to the elderly, who feel themselves restricted within their life and especially in the activity of the family or the things they love, such as working. This is the restriction of a mental concept. The mental concept of our world insists on "old age" as being a restricted life, and a restriction of the physical and mental activity of life. This mental concept creates restriction of the physical self. Change our mental image and we change our physical response which can help us to heal arthritis.

Whatever the restrictive force is, it is of the thinking mind first. The concept of restriction and oppression dictates decreased physical activity and a sedentary world. This creates a cycle of increased physical agony as our human body loses its freedom. As the restriction increases and the mind objects, the pain increases from the negative force of the thoughts. It becomes a self-perpetuated disease. Increased mental restriction increases the physical restriction which further restricts the mental condition, and on and on as the energy folds within itself.

This cycle must be consciously broken. Breaking the cycle of increased inactivity, pain and deformity is a lesson within itself. It requires the tremendous strength of singular focus. It requires diligent effort and tolerance of pain, as we loosen the restricted bands in our physical body and mind. In our physical world this is difficult perhaps to comprehend, but far from impossible when we choose to focus our thinking mind on the challenge that we face.

The perfect place to begin and to learn is with the cellular function. Many Souls suffering form arthritis eat large amounts of protein. The waste product of protein is urea. Urea can accumulate within the body and be the direct cause of physical pain and deformity. This can interfere with the assimilation of the organic mineral salts, even when we eat the foods of Nature. Many times these Souls do not eat the foods of Nature.

Arthritis is a disease of tremendous accumulation of waste matter within all systems of the physical self. To start the process of recovery requires the process of elimination of many foods from the diet, elimination of waste matter from the body, and elimination of oppression and restriction from the mind. This can best be accomplished by getting all thought out of the mind but freedom. Focus your meditation on freedom of body, mind, and Spirit. Focus your physical body on physical freedom by changing your diet to a cleansing diet of fruit. These should be citrus fruits – oranges, grapefruits, and the juice of limes and lemons. Eat nothing else for three days. Do not try to fast. This must be an eating process that will clean away the waste material. Eat all that you can eat and drink a minimum of ten glasses of pure water each day with lemon or lime juice added for additional cleansing. Ascorbic acid and the electromagnetic energy forces of the fruits of Nature are essential in this healing process. Never think that we can avoid the fruits and vegetables of Nature and overcome arthritis. Fruits and vegetables are our deficiency. Our excesses are fat and protein. Adjust your foods accordingly.

The thinking mind must be in coordination with the body for the healing to occur. We must know that we are being nourished to restore our body. We are not in physical danger. After a few days of cleansing, we will feel freer than we have felt in years. Focus your mind on your freedom of movement. Continue eating citrus fruits for a minimum of three days. If you feel hungry and crave food, add four raw non-starchy vegetables per day at lunch, and four steamed non-starchy vegetables for dinner.

These additional foods can be eaten from the beginning if hunger becomes an issue. Eat them in their natural state. Add only lemon juice or lime juice as seasoning. Eat all the quantity that you desire. This program should be continued for three to four weeks.

While eating in this manner you should begin a walking program, building it gradually based upon your own capabilities. Do not stress yourself but walk and breathe deeply of fresh air. Swimming is another exercise that should be enjoyed on a daily basis. Water is essential in the world of the arthritic. Soak in the tub, swim, and shower, do whatever is available to you, and do it frequently. While immersed in water, begin moving your joints gently, not forcing but simply moving. Keep your water comfortably warm while doing this, and be certain to have the body under water while moving. This is the ideal way to regain physical mobility.

Continue this program of exercise and eating for as long as necessary to restore the body. After four weeks the diet can be changed to the maintenance program in this book. Continue to eat protein sparingly. If you are hungry, increase the first generation foods. *Your body will respond to the love and care that you give it.* This care should be continued for a loving physical response, from the inner you. Avoid as much stress as possible, and change your lifestyle to be in a position to exercise total freedom of choice in who you are and who you want to be. Control can enhance our disease and we can end up being physically crippled.

Be a participant of life. Let the joyous, playful child out in the sun to play. Treat yourself to an indoor swimming pool or large tub to use several times a day. Keep the freedom of your body in rhythm with the freedom of your Spirit. Change, move forward, and celebrate life and living. Let the fear and restriction be in your past. Do not honor it with memory or concern. Persistent hydrotherapy will restore muscles, remove spurs and loosen tendons. All exercises should initially be done with your limbs underwater to avoid pain or further damage. Later, stretching exercises can be added if done gradually and gently. Try a television, online, or video class and stop when your body tells you to stop.

Any discussion of disease and any suggested therapeutic approach in this book is an attempt to show you what you can do, if you have the will to be well. It is not necessarily complete for each and every person because of the difference in Souls. If you are working with any of these lessons, you will need guidance and support. Ask for your own guidance from the Universe, or search for a practitioner to guide you.

Knowing that disease is of the mind, a created illusion to help you on your path of Soul evolution, is the first step to overcoming disease on the physical level. Restoring the physical body is usually possible, but it must be done with the will and intent of the mind, and it must be done gently and slowly until your body is used to the increased movement. It is your internal process; no one else can do it for you. Once we have established a strong intention within our mind and body coordination, it will require physical application to create the healing. There are many good teachers in our society that you can seek out and enjoy.

Heart and Blood Vessel Disease

Heart and blood vessel disease involves many diseases in our world. The term refers to all diseases of the heart and blood vessels as is indicated in the name. In our world these are many. The problems that occur in this system all occur for the same reasons of improper eating habits, lack of exercise, and the need for love. They may be manifested differently in each individual. When we eat the wrong foods our body suffers the consequences. When we fail to give love, we will stop receiving love. This is the Law of Compensation.

Knowing that all disease is, on the physical plane, the result of excesses and deficiencies of the foods that we eat, the lifestyle that we live, and the activity of the mind and body, we can clearly understand that the diseases of this system are no different. Knowing that the body is the direct result of the mind, the thoughts that we think and the beliefs that we hold, we can see that heart and blood vessel disease is indeed what we create. All disease is a lesson of the physical and as such no human lives and leaves this Earth without having created some physical dis-ease or disease.

The Soul that has evolved far enough to understand all of the lessons of the physical no longer incarnates into the human or Earth plane. There will always be lessons on Earth. Earth is the school for the Soul. Heart and blood vessel disease, more than any other disease, is a lesson in physical awareness of our self and our body. The heart and the blood vessels are the physical system of the life force of the physical self. They are the home of our blood and the electrical pumping system, which nourishes every cell within the entire cellular structure of our body. Without the oxygen, water and mineral salts, which our blood carries to the heart and other systems and cells, our body would die a physical death. The heart has the job of generating the electrical energy to pump this blood through the system of vessels, to nourish the body and to carry away the waste material. The activity of this system is essential to the continuation of our physical life. The goal of the physical body is survival.

We have been given the task of survival, to house the mind and Spirit within. The body is a product of the mind and Spirit. The viability of the heart and blood vessels dictates survival for this body. Therefore, this system will compromise other systems in the body, before it will compromise its own survival. This is seen in our world every day, when Souls with heart disease have multiple problems. The needs of the heart and blood vessels will create problems within other organs. This is normal in a body that is in the survival mode.

In our world, the medical profession frequently does blood tests. These blood tests will tell us sometimes that we are well when we are not well. The reason for this discrepancy in values is the survival process of the physical self. The blood will be the last place to indicate problems of the other cellular systems. Our human body is designed for survival. Blood is necessary for its survival. The alkaline-acid balance of the blood is necessary for survival. The viability of the blood will be maintained longer than the viability of any other cellular system. Understanding that this system of the body is going to be the last to show mineral deficiencies, for example, will allow us to understand that some systems of our body can be in serious condition before they will be medically apparent.

A common example of this is the *calcium deficiencies* that people have. Calcium deficiencies are known to occur under certain circumstances such as a decrease in estrogen production, increased age and with certain disease syndromes, but our world doesn't clearly understand how common calcium deficiency is in the creation of heart and blood vessel disease. It is not fully understood, because it is hard to scientifically prove by measurement of the blood calcium, which is not always accurate when the blood is drawn because of the normal fluctuation of the calcium levels.

Calcium is directly responsible for the contraction and relaxation of the heart and blood vessels. The body will continue to remove calcium from other cells of the body to maintain the calcium in the blood level. Calcium will be removed from the muscle, nerve, bone and all other cells to assure that the blood cells maintain their necessary balance. This is normal body function. This is survival for us which is built into our human design. This process repeats itself with every element needed to maintain the viability of the blood. The blood is the life force and therefore needs the elements of Nature for survival. It uses them, transports them and nourishes other cells with them.

Because of this process of need, the blood will take what it needs from wherever it is used or stored. This can create deficiencies in every other system within the body, if the needed elements are not continually being replaced and available to the blood from the digestive system. This leeching process, in itself, creates other diseases such as the collagen, muscle, mental and nerve diseases. These are our diseases of deficiencies that are compounded by our excesses. Excesses create deficiencies by the imbalance they create. Ingestion of an excess of improper food creates a deficiency of proper food. Deficiency of fibrous food creates an excess of waste material. Nothing within the body ever remains a singular action; it becomes a chain reaction impacting the entire body. This is the Universal Law of Cause and Effect.

This leeching process also creates its own heart and blood vessel disease, such as high blood pressure. Deficient mineral salts create a process that forces the blood to pump harder through the body to collect the elements it needs from other cells. This is an interference with the smooth and effortless flow of energy through the blood vessels. It is also increased work for the heart which can lead to heart disease.

Every action has a resulting reaction.

Excess fats will at the same time become an obstructive force within the blood vessels, causing a deficiency of blood flow. This obstruction requires excess pressure within the blood vessels, for the blood to pass through the vessels and on to the next system. This creates another link in the chain of problems and hard work for the blood vessels. The vessel itself needs calcium to continue its pulsation response to the beat of the heart. A deficiency in mineral salts causes a reaction of excess in the energy required to pump the blood through the vessels. As the vessels lose elasticity they no longer function as efficiently to move the blood through the system, and this decreased flow of energy increases the excess work of the heart, which leads many people directly into heart disease.

Another factor enters into the process of heart and blood vessel disease, which is the factor of excess. In our unaware state we eat what we think is good food. We have been told and shown how to eat since birth. We follow the belief that our knowledge is accurate. We are unaware of the creation of disease that we are producing within our body. And we are also unaware that we have as many versions of right and wrong in eating as we have people in the world. The intuitive mind knows on a Universal level that we are to eat from the foods of Nature. When the intellect or ego holds another belief, the mind itself is not in a state of balance. The rational mind and the intuitive mind as Universal minds are aware of the havoc the intellectual mind and the ego are creating within the physical self.

If we are unaware of the intuitive self or the rational self, we will be unaware that our mind is building according to our dictates and beliefs rather than in harmony with the laws of Nature. To complicate this problem, we will also be unaware on an intellectual level that the bulk of the information that we have been taught may not be accurate in this time and age. We will be unaware of the effects and the physical consequences of that inaccurate information. As a creation from Nature, we are always subject to the Laws of Nature despite our level of awareness. We cannot change this reality with our intellect.

As humans we eat large amounts of protein, fats, and salt, drink large amounts of soda with artificial sweetener or sugar, eat lots of sweets, drink many cups of coffee or tea, eat processed foods full of fats, sugars, and chemicals, drink alcohol or smoke cigarettes, and our behaviors frequently decrease the absorption of calcium and other mineral salts. If we are consuming all of the above, we may be consuming very few of Nature's foods. The foods of Nature are abundant with mineral salts that provide the electromagnetic energy forces that our body needs, and the other nutrients that we need to survive as human beings.

We eat with the intention of staying healthy. Our intellectual mind has been programmed with much false information. It is only through the lesson of awareness that we can learn to protect the credibility of our physical self on Earth. If we were all eating as we should eat, we would not have the intensity of diseases that we live with on a daily basis. All diseases have a basis in this lesson of awareness, just as all diseases are caused by excesses and deficiencies on the physical level. For those who are learning lessons of awareness, the choice of diseases will remain despite the advancement of their level of awareness. That does not mean that a Soul should not learn the lesson of awareness. Once awareness is learned then the choice is yours. If it is a lesson mastered it can help us overcome the disease, when we feel that lesson to be complete.

We Are What We Eat

Awareness is not mastery but it is one step forward in understanding healing the body with the mind.

A crucial factor in heart and blood vessel disease is total nutritional intake. We truly eat from the "tree of knowledge" rather than the trees of Nature. Our body is what we feed it. This is the Law of Cause and Effect. We are what we eat. We literally build our body by the food we provide it for the building process. We can only correct the creation by correcting the materials we use in the building. If we decided to build a house, a mansion, we would not go to the city dump and pick up junk of low quality to start building our mansion. If we bought junk, we would be building a shack, not a mansion. The shack that we build could have multiple problems. To build a mansion we would spend time choosing the materials carefully, selecting only high quality products and we would put them together creatively to build the mansion that is in our dreams.

As human beings, we follow this pattern consistently for our physical house, so that we can live in comfort and peace, enjoying the luxury of the protection that our house gives us. We will furnish it lovingly, buying the best in decorations, painting, papering, and constantly caring for our creation. We will shower it with love and attention, giving it the best. Our physical body is a house. It is the house of the mind and Spirit. It is the physical shelter that we give our eternal self as human beings on Earth. We build it block by block, cell by cell. We create the body in which our mind and Spirit will be required to function. We create the balance or imbalance within our own human bodies.

We are totally responsible for what we build. Build your body from the best in materials and put them together lovingly and creatively. Lavish your house with love and attention. Allow it the freedom of love and inner peace. This is the balance which we create when we create a mansion of self. We must understand that we build by our actions and we must accept the responsibility for what we build. This is awareness. If we take materials from the city dump and we slap them together with anger and hate, we will have a house that is tumbling down. We will have a physical body that lives in fear and physical pain. We will create an internal imbalance of the mind and Spirit, which will result in disease.

For those Souls who are learning the lesson of awareness, there is hope. As long as the Spirit continues to reside within the physical self, we have the power to create health. The Spirit is the inspiration and motivation of life. The Spirit is the will and intention to live and to do what needs to be done, to learn the lesson that we are teaching ourselves. The motivation of life is allowing the Spirit freedom to love and to BE, the mind freedom to build a healthy body, and providing the physical materials the body needs to proceed.

The cleansing program will rid our body of waste material. Nature's foods will restore our physical balance.

The Spirit of life will give us the intention and the will to lavish our house with love and caring for ourselves and others. For those Souls with heart and blood vessel disease, exercise is a necessity of life. Exercise increases the flow of blood through the heart and blood vessels to nourish every organ and cell within the body. It increases the circulation of all systems. Sitting will pool blood within the vessels, and present blockage and the increased need for force within the vessel, if our blood vessels are abnormal.

Use it or Lose it!

What the body finds we are not using, it will by nature inactivate. If we want our body to be in good condition, we must use it. This applies to all parts of the physical self. If we want to keep an active mind, we must continue to use it. If we want an active sex life, we must continue to have sex. What the body does not use, it shuts down. The mind controls the body. If the mind is not focused on using the body or any part of the body, it sends an unconscious message to that part of the self. This message of the mind will result in a decreased blood flow to that part of the body, which will compromise the function of the body part. These issues can be frequently found in people with heart disease.

The most important lesson for us in the concept of disease is awareness of how we are living our life. Be aware of what you are doing to your body. Be aware of the control, the influence your mind and thoughts have on your physical body. Understand that in every moment of living, you are in the business of creation. This is not simply the creation of your physical world; it is the creation of the physical self and your relationship to the physical world.

We do not move one muscle of our body without producing a reaction someplace else in our body. We do not eat one bite of food that does not produce multiple reactions within our physical self. We do not walk without producing multiple reactions within our physical self. We do not even think, no matter what the subject, without creating an internal response within our physical self. We do not see or hear without creating an internal response. This helps us to understand the concept of "always think positive thoughts." Understanding that we are our own creation will allow us to choose wisely in the creating. Knowing that each and every exposure to all that is around us, all that we think, all that we eat, all that we do, is the building material of our individual creation allows us the freedom of choice. It is in exercising this choice that we produce disease, fear, anger, hate and unhappiness or we can produce vibrant health, longevity, joy, happiness, peace and love. It is our choice.

Understanding that all of life is a choice will allow us to understand that we have the capability to overcome disease if we have it. Healing ourselves will require a change in lifestyle, a change in eating habits, a change in attitude and a change in our belief system. It will require that we love ourselves, and the Universe that is Spirit's creation.

Awareness of the reaction we create within our body will help us choose the action that we wish to experience. We may have to evaluate our life, our thoughts and our food to understand the action that precipitated a reaction, but if the desire is there to understand, we will understand.

Each and every disease known to us is a reaction of our action. Every disease we know can be healed, if we want to be healed. We will not cover other diseases here because this book is intended to help you with your awareness of cause and effect as we live it physically. The book is written as an overview to trigger your awareness. An awareness of cause gives us the power to heal ourselves of all disease, if it is our will to do so. Healing does not include healing the trauma of deformity, because that is its own lesson that was accepted for this lifetime on Earth by the Dual Soul.

An awareness of cause as it relates to us and our lives can allow us to live the Joy of Health. The balance of body, mind, and Spirit will protect us from disease, and create the experience of a long and productive lifetime on this Earth level. Live in peace and joy, and you will live in the joy of health.

OUR RESPONSIBILITY

FRESH AIR, PURE WATER, FOODS OF NATURE

Maintaining the health of our body with the proper foods does not mean that we have to give up eating. That would be counter-productive to health and happiness. Since our cellular structure is determined by the components we give our body, we need to look at what that responsibility means for each of us from a practical viewpoint.

Eating correctly from only healthy foods is our number one responsibility. What we put into our bodies and how our bodies handle what we provide is the primary issue. In the Book that we call the Bible, Genesis tells us that Spirit made man from the Earth. That is a symbolic statement which indicates we are an integrated part of Nature. Our physical bodies are made of the exact elements that are found as elements of the Earth. Life depletes the bodily resources, and our responsibility is replenishing those resources in their natural form, which will keep our human body chemically balanced and healthy.

We are responsible for providing our bodies with the elements it needs for the survival of our cellular structure and function. Those elements are FRESH AIR, PURE WATER, and the FOODS OF NATURE. Our body has been designed to take in air and let out a gas, which is the waste material produced by the body's utilization of oxygen. This happens automatically. To stop breathing is to stop life. Our breathing is automatic because it is crucial to life. Earth is designed with the air that we need in exactly the correct and necessary mixture of oxygen and nitrogen that the body requires for living.

We are responsible for the way that we breathe. We need to fill our lungs completely with air, to provide the proper amount of gases to the blood and tissue to create our physical self. We are responsible for maintaining the purity of the air of our world. We are responsible for the pollution of our lungs; if we smoke or inhale other gases or chemicals intentionally or knowingly, we can damage our lungs. These are our responsibilities as human beings in maintaining the quality of the air we breathe automatically.

Water is the next element that is essential to our human life. We can live only minutes without air. We can live only hours without water. In human form, we are primarily water. Water is essential to the function and life of every cell in our body. Spirit made fruits and vegetables to contain large amounts of water. This was the way of protecting the human body as we began life on Earth.

The conscious use of water becomes our responsibility in maintaining our physical health. Once we accept personal responsibility for the internal process of breathing as essential to our physical existence, our cellular function will continue automatically. Water is held in disdain by many in our world. It is ignored, polluted, and undervalued. Water is the best and purest medicine in our Universe. The healing properties of water have been recognized from the beginning of our human culture. But in our present culture, water healing is seldom used. Water can be used to cure many diseases, to give physical and emotional comfort, to provide vitality, and to prevent aging and disease. It is Spirit's elixir. Spirit made water necessary and available for the essential act of living.

Water should be consumed in its purest state and consumed frequently during the day. It flushes waste material from the body and cleanses the cells. The food we eat presents the various systems of the body with large amounts of waste matter. It is this waste matter that causes many of our diseases of excess. Without water, we would harbor these diseases constantly within our human design. When we consistently consume the proper amount of water we can avoid many diseases.

Water should be used externally to cleanse the body. Soaking in water maintains the fluid balance internally and the correct balance of organisms externally. Many of our diseases have been and are diseases of filth. Without daily bathing, the external organisms multiply and can be absorbed into the skin through the pores, resulting in disease. When our body's fluid balance is not maintained, the body becomes more susceptible to disease.

It is our responsibility to provide our body with water internally and externally. We can learn to calm our body and our mind with little effort and much joy, simply by using the water that Spirit has made plentiful on Earth. The Universe continues to send us more as we need it.

Accepting our responsibility for the use of water in our daily lives frees us to go about our daily dramas with little concern for the viability of the cells within us. This is a simple task for us and relieves us of many physical concerns. Our body is designed to function automatically if it is taken care of properly. It will function automatically, if we supply it with the air, water and the natural food that it requires. Consuming foods that are free of any man-made sprays and other chemicals is absolutely critical for a healthy body.

The next elements that Spirit designed as essential to the function of the physical self were put into the plants that were placed upon the Earth. Within the plants of the Earth is every element that will assure our body of physical health and chemical balance upon Earth. There is nothing else necessary for the health of the physical body, if we use the air we breathe, the water of the Earth and the plants of the Earth for food. These elements fulfill the replenishing of chemicals within our body that we lose in living. Cancer is showing us that we are failing to replenish our body with the chemicals that it needs, but we are putting chemicals into our body that our body cannot cope with on a daily basis.

"Garbage In, Garbage Out"

Using plant foods in their natural form will prevent disease. The electromagnetic energy force that is in the foods of Nature can supply us with the chemical deficiencies that now cause disease. These electro-magnetic energy forces are partially recognized in our world as mineral salts. These salts will help remove the excesses that cause disease and they will balance out the deficiencies. These foods of Nature can cleanse and restore our physical body.

One of the lessons of life is learning to accept total responsibility for the physical body, thinking mind, and Spirit Senses. Accepting this responsibility requires that we provide our body with the elements needed to preserve the viability of the cells and maintain cellular structure and function. A familiar phrase of our society describes this problem as it occurs in our world. "Garbage in, garbage out." If we desire perfect function, it becomes our responsibility to provide the perfect elements of function for our body to use.

Since we are made from the elements of Nature, it is logical to assume that we must replace those elements of Nature as our body uses them in its daily function. We would not put beer into the gas tank of our car. We know that our car runs efficiently on the fuel its engine is designed to use for optimum performance, and we know that it only lasts a calculated number of miles before it needs to be replaced. We also know that if we put high-octane fuel in our car's gas tank, the engine will run longer. Our body can also be destroyed when we fill it with foreign chemicals. These chemicals create diseases that can be fatal.

We accept the responsibility of maintaining and repairing our physical toys more quickly and logically than we accept the responsibility for repairing our physical self. We will lavish loving care on our house, our car, our boat, and all of our physical possessions, but we will abuse our body on a daily basis and not be concerned. The mentality of our world is that our physician is responsible for our health. We are very quick to take an abused body to the physician, and complain that the physician failed to create the miracle of health. It is not the physician's responsibility. We are responsible for creating the health of our body, thinking mind, emotional self, and sensory self.

If we took our car to the shop in the exact state of disrepair that our body is in when we go to a physician, the mechanic would tell us to junk the car. If a physician told us that our body was beyond repair, we would blame the physician for not being able to fix it. No matter what a physician does to help us, he or she cannot live our life for us. He cannot be with us minute by minute of each and every day, to be sure that we eat what we should eat, exercise, stop smoking, and stop drinking. Those responsibilities belong to each of us. They cannot be given to another person, no matter who that person is.

Today's physicians have been taught to treat disease. They do this in the manner in which they have been taught. They were not taught to perform "miracles" in medical school. This can be compared to blaming a train wreck on the train. We are the engineers of our physical, mental, sensory, and emotional health because it is our everyday reality. The health of our physical body and the life that we live are the result of how we think, what we do, and our belief system. There is nowhere else to place the responsibility for living a life of health, except with the individual whose body and life it is.

Health is not a miracle, it is a personal responsibility. The joy and freedom that good health gives us creates the miracle of a good and long life. When Spirit designed us, She created a miracle. That miracle can continue to be a miracle, if we simply fulfill our daily maintenance responsibility. Once our personal abuse has become a habit or an addiction, it requires our intent and will to restore the physical to its miracle state of functioning. The physician alone cannot do this. He can offer us guidance and help us, but the responsibility for the doing is ours.

Eating the fruits, vegetables, nuts, seeds and grains from Nature's bounty is a true joy for both our body and Soul. When we eat these foods, an interesting thing will begin to happen within our body. A change will occur very quickly in our body's cravings and tastes. Normally three to seven days will be enough to become aware of the change. During this time we must eat only natural food and drink pure water, to notice the effect. Nature's food will begin to taste sweet and nourishing to our body. Eating fresh foods will give us joy.

This will work even for those of us that "hate" the foods of Nature. If we are interested in health, it is worth trying. The foods of Nature restore all of the chemicals that make up our human design and put our physical body, mind, and Spirit back into the precise chemical balance that we are designed to have. Processed foods will become tasteless, as we miss the natural flavor of the mineral salts that are plentiful in the natural world of food. The digestion and assimilation of the natural food gives us a burst of energy that we may not have felt in years.

We are providing our body with the elements necessary for cellular health and function. When our body is functioning perfectly, our mind will function perfectly. We will feel ourselves bursting with the internal energy of life and happiness. We may begin to believe that a miracle has occurred. Our cellular energy increases our normal physical senses. We will find ourselves conscious of tastes, smells, sounds, and visual images that we were never conscious of before. We will begin to feel by touch, sense, and knowing the "energy" of the people around us.

Removing the garbage from your body removes the compromised condition of function that the cells have known. Compromising the function that the cellular activity presents to the physical body with an electrical deficiency that dulls the physical response is the very beginning of making ourselves sick. We have five physical senses: seeing, hearing, smelling, tasting, touching. We also have a supreme physical sense which is the combination of the five physical senses being used at any one time. This supreme physical sense is the sexual response.

Why have less than "perfect sex"?

When we eat improperly, we block some or all of our physical senses. How many people do you know who say, "I can't smell anything," or "I can't taste anything"? These people are abusing their bodies and they are blocking their five physical senses. If any one of the five physical senses is blocked, the supreme physical response that we call sex is less than perfect. Increasing cellular activity can be compared to putting a new cartridge in our printer or a new ink cartridge in our fountain pen. Suddenly the print becomes clear again. Suddenly, sexual activity becomes great again.

With improper elements for cellular function, the cells will spend excessive energy on survival for the body. This is the functioning level for many bodies in our world. Dis-ease is indeed survival, it is not vital living. The organic mineral salts that plant foods provide for our cells act as the conductors and generators of energy currents within the cells. Without them we have a decrease in the physical, mental, emotional, and Spiritual energy that we feel, and that we can use in our daily lives. Understand that whatever level of physical life that we are living, we can live more efficiently if we accept the responsibility for change.

Before the mechanical revolution, physical bodies became acclimated to the foods grown from the soil on which they lived. They moved as the weather changed, because they were responsible for providing the food they needed to eat. They had fewer diseases of malnutrition than we have today. Now we have become a nomadic society again but in a different way. We have access to all of Nature's foods from our corner grocery store. When we accept the responsibility of choice in what we eat, we can get the proper elements of Nature without moving.

Nearly seventy years ago when our society developed the World War II mentality, or commercial mentality in relationship to food, we created increased health problems. The commercial mentality simply built more laboratories, made more new drugs, processed more food with chemicals, and built more hospitals. Today's senior citizens are basically a generation that ate differently. Because they ate differently, they have the potential to restore their bodies, if they can change their belief system. The present generation may not become senior citizens without some conscious changes in their eating habits and lifestyle. It is fortunate that many people today are developing an awareness of the needs of their physical bodies. These are the true "teachers" of the world that are on Earth to teach the masses. Teachers are also leaders.

True Teachers are also Leaders

Those children born into this commercial mentality are the ones we want to teach. Their parents will understand and they can help. The commercial mentality demands instant gratification. Today our health problems are extreme and they demand instant cures. Our personal responsibility for life and our health is many times not recognized and accepted. It is time for us to look within. Children and adults with this "commercial" mentality have chosen a self-destructive course. The relationship between a fast-food culture and a drug culture is apparent.

Everything in our world is geared toward self-gratification and self-aggrandizement. There must be someone to accept the blame. There must be someone that can provide instant gratification. There must be something that can make us happy. There must be something that can be eaten at once and without work. This is the commercial mentality at work. It has become an accepted culture and a coveted culture. It is also a destructive culture for the physical body, and it is without peace and happiness for the mind. Truly there is no one but you to be responsible for you and to acknowledge the responsibility for yourself.

The perspective for all of life is learning a lesson. Each Soul will return again and again until the lesson of the physical is understood and lived. *The true basis of the human being is energy.* Energy never dies but it does change form, which has been proven by Albert Einstein. Learning to balance our physical body as energy and matter is a Dual Soul lesson. Learning to accept responsibility is a personal lesson. There is no wrong. There is only action and reaction. The total responsibility for every human being is accepting responsibility for self.

We cannot seek balance externally from another person and expect that balance to last indefinitely. Our human balance comes from our human energy and our energy must come from within the body, mind, and Spirit of each individual. Accepting personal responsibility is knowing and accepting that we alone are responsible for the reality we create, whether it is of the physical, the mental, or the Spiritual. There is no one else to blame. Life is our many lessons in personal responsibility that begins with our physical self, expands into our mental and emotional self, and then expands into our sensory self as the design of our Spiritual self.

Accepting personal responsibility for eating correctly, breathing deeply, drinking water in adequate quantities, exercising our body and keeping loving thoughts within our mind belongs to each human being and it must be learned as we live different lifetimes. We can always tell the advancement of our Dual Soul by the behavior that we live. When we accept our individual responsibility for self, we will in turn accept our responsibility for the Earth that provides our energy and our balance. We will recognize the rhythm as being the rhythm of Nature. We will be inviting the inner peace of health into our daily world.

ADDICTIONS

Addiction in our world is more excessive than we realize. It is a sad plight for us because we cannot acknowledge that we have an addictive problem that is affecting our personality and our behavior. We do not think of ourselves as being sick. We do not recognize that addiction is a disease. Addiction is an illusion of "need" for the ego. It is the illusion that is coveted. It will take an addict years to acknowledge his or her problem, and years longer, perhaps, to seek treatment. And it may take many years longer before the addict can heal his/her addictions.

Illusions are difficult to identify because they are not physical in our physical world. *An illusion is a false belief.* We may attempt to accept our addictions as our illusions, but this shows us that we are also living and learning the lesson of addictions in our physical reality. Addiction can be physical, psychological, mental, behavioral, emotional or religious. Illusions cover all realms of our physical reality. The need is there, but it isn't there. It is the belief and behaviors that make addictions a reality in our terms. There are no empty spaces in the Universe.

Addiction is known by other names such as habit, love, cravings, need, desire, wants, and various other terms. Anytime that we have a behavior that we feel we cannot live without, we are addicted to the behavior. All addictions are the result of the belief system that we have been involved with from the beginning of our life. The basic cause of addiction is the fear of separation from Spirit, which is our supreme illusion. What Spirit has created cannot be separated from Spirit or us as Spirit. Spirit is energy and we are energy.

We will see the fear of separation manifested in many different ways in the physical realm. Each and every manifestation is an attachment to a false belief. All attachments are ego attachments. Addictions vary in degree and in importance. The cause of the addiction is more important than the addiction itself. It is important to search for an understanding of our illusion about any addiction. If the physical manifestation of cause is not apparent, the addiction should be dealt with from the concept of root cause, which is always the fear of separation from Spirit that is seldom recognized.

Addictions may start with a need in one system such as the body and progress to a mental and emotional need as well. The progression and the regression of any addiction are controlled by the individual and his belief system. We must change the belief system to successfully treat the disease. Belief is an illusion of the ego. It has no true physical reality. All addictions affect the health and happiness that a Soul experiences. An addiction can destroy our physical life, our friends, and our career. Even lesser addictions are hard for others to observe in the one they love.

Addiction is the opposite of freedom and all addictions acknowledge an attachment to fear that is a resistance to change. Resisting change is resisting growth. This is the ego action of attachment to the illusion. Addiction, in any form, is a reaction to some facet of our being that holds us captured in fear. It can be the reaction to a combination of fears or beliefs that occurred at another moment in our life that has created our addictions. At this moment in our life we may no longer fear the same thing, but this addiction energy creates a need through the mind attachment which we are resisting changing in our present reality. When we fear change we allow events, thoughts, beliefs, and other activities to hold us captive.

Addiction can be defined in our terms as a fear reaction of physical, mental, and emotional resistance to change. Let us use an example to clarify this statement. In high school you may have found yourself feeling shy and insecure around the other students. You may have felt them to be more beautiful, more handsome, more intelligent, more prosperous, and more athletic or many other "mores" than you were. They may have all developed the habit of smoking. You felt too insecure not to join them. You were afraid that if you didn't conform to what your friends were doing, you would be separated from the friendships. You would be cast out, so to speak, because you were different. This fear of rejection developed your habit of smoking. It all started from a tiny fear that was controlling your thinking.

Today you feel that you would not be "comfortable" in a crowd, unless you smoked. That cigarette, which gave you security as a teenager, is still giving you security. You are mentally still attached to the illusion of need. It is still helping you deal with the fear of separation. If you didn't smoke, you would have to talk to people. You couldn't think if you couldn't take a long drag on the cigarette. You would have to answer immediately and you might not know the answer. See how the ego self works? The ego fears that it would not be good enough, it would not be worthy, without a prop. The ego fears separation from the security of the cigarette. You are being controlled by the cigarette. Where is your strength?

Do you see the fear of separation that this presents to the ego? Do you see the illusion of unworthiness that you are attached to? Do you see that you do not love yourself by clinging to this belief? In this book we will deal with our fear addictions in the way of an overview, because our addictions control us, our world, our relationships, and our careers. Our world is created by our multiple illusions of fear. When this fear is reacted to through addictions, it has become an ego-controlling fear. Therefore, the subject is too expansive and too common to discuss adequately in one short commentary. But we cannot live the joy of health and at the same time be totally controlled by and addicted to our fears, which we choose to act out by using substances that threaten our health and happiness.

We have many addictions that fall within the category of common and accepted use, such as: alcohol, tobacco, food, drugs, sex, gambling, eating, status, relationships, and many others. We will speak of only a few of these. Addiction to foods and chemicals is extremely common on Earth. The substance the body craves the most is the substance it usually needs the least, but has developed an addiction to. Addiction occurs from excessive use or attachment. All addiction is caused by this fear that is being caused by an imbalance in our body, mind, and Spirit. When the body is balanced it has no cravings. It is balanced. Addiction is an imbalance. Addiction is always some form of excessive thinking or behavior focused on a belief, or something in particular such as a chemical or a behavior.

The only true cure for addiction is a Spiritual Awakening.

Addiction occurs primarily in people who have focused their growth or energy within either the physical or mental facets of self. These people will have totally or partially denied the Spiritual self. An acknowledgement of the Spirit will balance the human trilocular self and remove the craving, the attachment that we have created to the physical world around us. There is a fluidity to the energy forces within the body that flow smoothly with the peace of balance. When one part of the body, mind, and Spirit is denied, the body is captured within a lopsided energy imbalance that produces extreme cravings. This imbalance is so critical that each time the energy flows through the body the body feels the loss of balance and turns to an addiction or addictive substance for its image of survival.

Addiction becomes a behavioral pattern within our life. We could be said to develop an "addictive personality." This is a self-destructive, multi-addictive approach to life which happens when we are in total Spiritual denial. We create more and more addictions because we identify them with a way to balance ourselves and to understand life better. This is the ultimate in illusions. This person will have an energy flow that has lumps, bumps, branches, crevices and other irregularities impeding the rhythm. This is a sick and destructive energy that will need a Spiritual awakening to provide the physical strength to cure itself.

An addictive personality focuses on a few addictions to the excess and the exclusion of all else. This is very common with drug, alcohol, and food addicts. When the body does not receive the elements it needs it will accept the substitutes of the mind cravings. It has no choice. The body is on a downhill slide and it will eventually break down internally and externally. It will become desperate in its need unless we recognize that we have the power to control our addictive energy.

The body is built by the mind, and when deprived of the essential elements it must accept second best. The body has become programmed to survive temporarily in that mode of operation. If the mind is captured in fear and the body has learned to release that fear with a substance, the body will demand the substance. *The goal of the physical body is survival.* The human body will do its best to survive, under the most bizarre circumstances that we can create with our boundless imagination.

This marvelous cellular structure that we call a body can literally make a new person out of us with our cooperation and motivation of life. All the body is searching for is balance. The most common food addictions in our world are fats, sugars, starches and salt. The most common chemical addictions are alcohol, nicotine, food preservatives, tranquilizers, pain pills, and sleeping pills. The most commonly accepted drug addictions are laxatives, anti-acids, cough syrups, decongestants, vitamins, and minerals. We have created a "pill-centered" society which holds us captive in our image of "poor health."

These addictions are not acknowledged by our society except for a partial acknowledgement of the chemical addictions. The unacknowledged addictions are greater in number because of the unawareness of the potential for harm. We do not realize that any substance that is used excessively on a regular basis can create a behavioral and psychological addiction. The physical reaction will be different from the body's reaction to a serious drug such as cocaine, but there will be a reaction. Addiction does not mean that the substance itself is wrong and should never be used. Addiction means that the use of the substance is out of control by the individual and it is used with the wrong intention.

When we use a substance or food in an addictive manner, the body will reprogram itself to accept that substance as "the substance that is needed." Therefore, the body will trigger the craving to avoid depletion. A substance that is "filling in" for what the body really needs is needed in larger and larger amounts for attempted conversion to the natural elements of Nature. The physical need for the substitute will increase as the essential elements decrease within the body. A substance that has virtually no food value causes a progressive state of physical imbalance. Physical imbalance leads to mental and emotional imbalance. Physical and mental imbalance lead to a Spiritual imbalance or this energy can acknowledge awareness and create a Spiritual search.

The cells in the body will utilize all of the stored elements. The body will work overtime in its attempt to convert other chemicals to the needed elements. As the viability of the cells decreases, there will be a decrease in the absorption of other nutrients and a decrease in body elimination. The poisons that are created require more in an environment of less. This imbalance that has been created is common and is one of the primary causes of disease in our society.

An example of this type of addiction is someone who craves chocolate. Our little addict eats nothing but chocolate all day long. If other foods are added, they are usually other sugars or starches. They all have no true food value. They have no electromagnetic energy to provide. This addiction will cause severe obesity, malnutrition with liver damage, constipation, high blood pressure, and a multitude of other physical complaints. There is heaviness to the Soul of this person, because there is no joy in her life. She has created disease from her addiction to chocolate. There are Souls that have chosen this method to leave Earth, without staying to learn the lessons of the physical life.

This drama of addiction results in many complicated medical problems. Many of these problems are generated because of a lack of awareness in the person and within the medical community. It is important that we all begin to fully understand that all excesses create deficiencies. This is especially true in the area of nutrition, but it is also true in all of life. We are searching for balance. Dietary deficiencies are not something that can be easily accepted and therefore they are not easily corrected, which allows the life of that person to begin the slide into oblivion and death.

Is it logical that we are living in the land of plenty and can suffer from malnutrition? Our body can do a commendable job of creation, but we must give it the tools to work with. Many instances of disease are the direct result of our chemical deficiencies, which are created by our excesses. Headaches, which are common, are a disease of deficiency and excess. Depression is a disease that is also created by both excesses and deficiencies without most people understanding this relationship. This helps us to understand how important it is for us to develop an awareness of self.

Addictions and Allergies

Addictions to some foods will create what we call allergic reactions to these foods. This allergic reaction will be manifested by the creation of supposedly unrelated diseases. For instance, an abundance of sugar in the diet can create an allergic reaction that triggers arthritis, headaches, hyperactivity, depression, infections and a host of other problems. Milk and ice cream can cause severe asthma. This too, is known as an allergic reaction. The allergic reaction will occur secondary to excessive or addictive use of the food that we are allergic to. The chemicals added to foods exacerbate the reactions we have as we expand our internal imbalance.

At this point of addiction we will not feel well because we are becoming totally unbalanced. We are as desperate on the inside on a cellular level as we are on the outside on every physical level. We are indeed unbalanced! This drama of addiction results in many complicated medical problems that generally go unrecognized. Keep in mind that these addictions develop because of the fear of separation. Why was the chocolate addict trying to hide her beautiful figure? Was she afraid of men? Was she feeling unworthy and choosing to create her version of unworthiness? Why was the ice cream addict creating asthma? Did she feel smothered and fearful for her life? Do you see the dramas that we can create with addictions?

Admitting that we create our physical, intellectual, emotional, and sensory reality on a daily basis by our actions and thoughts, which are products of our belief system, will help us overcome this drama. It will put us in the position of accepting responsibility and control for who and what we are. When we can accept ourselves for who we are, we will have nothing to fear. We will find value and joy in being the "me" that we know.

Who Are We Hiding From?

Seeking treatment in our medical establishments for problems resulting from addictions and being treated with drugs and chemicals is the perfect way to compound the problem, not solve it. Drug therapy results in a serious depletion of the electromagnetic energy that promotes our cellular function and viability. The belief system of our society makes drugs not only accepted but coveted as a relief from personal responsibility for our physical and emotional well-being. Who are we hiding from? When we attempt to hide it is always from ourselves, because the rest of the world does not have any conscious investment in how badly or how often we screw up.

This leads a Soul on the path of least resistance and total cellular destruction. Drugs are often responsible for death in patients that found this their path of choice for leaving this incarnation. An addictive personality will take anything that is given to them. This is a lesson in personal responsibility. Only the Soul itself is responsible for the outcome of life. All of life is a choice. A serious addiction in our society is the addiction to alcohol and drugs. Those Souls who are captured in this addictive process are those who fear life the most. They may have everything in terms of material possessions, but in their hearts they are totally alone. There is a subconscious understanding that if they stay with alcohol and drugs, they will not ever have to accept the responsibility of love.

These are Souls who have intense fears of not being loved, of being separated from someone they love. In their emotional state, they will identify the one they are fearful of losing with a name. Names are unimportant. These are the people who feel the separation from Spirit Consciousness intensely. Remember that we are made in the image of Spirit as energy beings. Fear of separation from Spirit is a fear of the recognition of self. These Souls are intensely captured in their fear of self, their search for self. Many of them appear to the world as totally self-focused, selfish Souls. They ARE, in terms of the physical world. They are so fiercely caught up in this magnified fear that they can feel no love for themselves or anyone else.

This does not mean that they have no attachments. Remember, they have addictive personalities. Their attachment is the ego attachment of the "I" of self. It is not love of another person. If they can't love themselves, how could Spirit love them? They are sinners, drunks and liars, so how could Spirit love them? There really isn't a Spirit anyway, so does it really matter? These are the concepts that run through the mind of a person with an addictive personality. These thoughts are not only floating around in the subconscious, but they are in the conscious mind, too. They are conscious of every sinful moment that they have ever created in their life. There is a tug of war in this person between the ego and the Soul that few people would believe. It is a war of sin, guilt, unworthiness, and the denial of Spirit that would put a ship pirate to shame. A ship pirate would not worry about being good. That is not his lesson of the moment. But he would be worried about being forgiven when he was going to make his next "seizure" to keep his business going strong.

Our alcoholic is the classic cross between a devil and saint. He is bad, even when he isn't drunk, and he cringes in fear over the "mean old Spirit" who is looking over his shoulder. He denies, he resists, he won't change, he hates himself, he is usually uncomfortable around lots of people, he is a loner, he is lonely, he is charming and he is loveable. He is terrified that he will be separated from Spirit because of his behavior, but he is living in so much fear that he can't find the motivation to change. His normal comment would be: "It's too late now to worry about it. There really isn't a Spirit anyway. Let's have another drink."

The only true cure for addiction is a Spiritual Awakening.

We have said this before but we will repeat it here, because this is especially true when we are addicted to alcohol. Our addiction is rooted in our fear of separation from Spirit. Alcoholics have had a love, hate relationship with Spirit for their entire life. Many have spent time denying Spirit. A Spiritual Awakening gives the alcoholic the opportunity to see Spirit with a little different perspective.

Let me emphasize here the difference between a religious path and a Spiritual path. Religion has as its basis a fear of Spirit. Spiritualism has as its basis a love of Spirit. A religious path will increase the problems for most alcoholics, although this will depend on their individual perspective of Spirit. All addictions are created because of the fear of separation from Spirit. Love is the elixir that can solve many problems. Love offered in unison with a physical restoration program that is based on Nature's foods can soon restore the physical body to a non-addictive healthy state. This can be done in a period of weeks.

The months and years that we now struggle through life to overcome addiction are not essential to curing ourselves if the approach is balanced between our body, mind and Spirit. Identifying the basis of an addiction emotionally and replacing the cellular elements that will restore our physical body can accomplish a complete cure. The secret to this awareness of cause is looking within. The answer is never outside of us as human beings. The love that cures is the love of self, the Spirit self, not the ego self. Knowing that we are perfect within our Spirit self allows us to accept personal responsibility for that self. We can then know and act upon the love, the miracle that we are.

Life is the Ultimate in a Beautiful Chain.

Providing the right foods to protect the physical temple of that Spirit self then becomes our desire and our behavior. We are in control. Loving ourselves allows us to love other people. This could be compared to the most creative jeweler designing the ultimate in beautiful chains. Life is the ultimate in a beautiful chain. Each link grows from the last beautiful link until we have an unbroken circle of beauty. Within that chain of family and friends who love us is strength to break the fear of separation and enhance the beauty of our creation.

Loving an alcoholic, or loving a self-aholic, is a difficult and addictive behavior that mirrors the behavior of the alcoholic. Often these definitions are synonymous.

The alcoholic is always a self-aholic. Not all self-aholics are alcoholics, although the potential to create this addiction is prominent within. It may appear to some that the alcoholic that sleeps on the street and begs a bottle of wine could not possibly be a self-aholic. When there is love between two people, one of normal activity and one of alcoholic activity, the need to save develops in the non-drinker. The alcoholic is an addictive personality who has learned to control his world by role-playing, manipulation, charm, magnified need and singular self-focus. The alcoholic does not love himself/herself or he/she would not be captured in addictive behavior. Not loving ourselves requires that we focus full attention on ourselves to survive. Love is equal to trust and truth. If we fail to love ourselves we cannot trust ourselves or anyone else, and we cannot see truth in our world. Our alcoholic lives in the world of the alcoholic perspective. Nothing is truly real except our fear of separation which does not exist as a conscious fear.

This fear of separation will be from people, material possessions, jobs, etc. What we fear most will surely happen, because we do not have an investment in relationships. We have an investment, an acknowledgement in fear and self. We are very needy, we are very manipulative, and we are more than willing to play the role that indulges self. We will suffer a multitude of separations before we will truly look at ourselves with discernment. That self, which we are protecting so intensely, is the only life line that our subconscious self sees to Spirit. Acknowledging the self, the identity of self, is the acknowledgement of Spirit as our savior. Our alcoholic doesn't believe in Spirit, he believes in self. Do you see the vicious cycle that has been created within the mind of the alcoholic? Do you see the tug of war that is taking place between the Soul and the ego of our alcoholic?

What is happening to the people in our alcoholic friend's life? The ones who love him most, that try the hardest to help him with a vision of reality, are the ones who begin to mirror the behavior. This image becomes the addictive behavior of the savior. The savior will accept the stones, the insults, the loss of respect, the manipulative behavior that is self-depreciating to them, in their need to be the savior. These relationships become cycles of destructive behavior. Both parties in the relationship are captured in this negative energy flow.

True Value

There is no value to the relationship, because there is no value to the self. There is no appreciation from the alcoholic for the savior's attempts to support, encourage, and love. It is accepted and needed but it is not respected or appreciated. Love is not returned with love, because there is no love. There is only the "tug of war" that is eternal within the Soul and ego of the alcoholic. Value is not a word that is understood by the alcoholic. When two people are involved in this destructive cycle of illusion of need, it will continue until the savior can see the folly of it all and end the relationship.

The alcoholic never ends the relationships directly, because he is captured by his fear of separation. He ends all relationships through his self-focused, addictive actions which are then able to create the fear as a reality within his world. The alcoholic is in his own struggle and will usually stay in the illusion of need for thousands of incarnations. Only the Spiritual Awakening can restore the balance to the energy flow of this Soul.

The self-aholic is the person that focuses only on self, again for survival and the fear of separation from what he terms his identity. This identity is usually focused on the material. It may be a spouse, a job, material possessions or a combination of "things" that afford identification within the physical world. The self-aholic will covet other women or men as a means of self-flattery, self-involvement, self-love, and self-appreciation. He will covet women as the alcoholic covets alcohol. It will not be within his emotional or psychological capability to ever leave his "identity" for a relationship. His internal tug of war is the same as the alcoholic experience. The self-aholic defines self as his intellect. He functions from the ego level with a basic denial of the Spiritual level of self.

The self-aholic's behavior and his illusion of need will be the same as the alcoholic. His relationships will be depreciating because of his lack of acknowledgement and commitment. They are, in his mind, another possession. They are based on self-infatuation not love of another person. We have no pre-determination for disease, addiction or deterioration. We have the choice to be what we want to be. When we make the choice not to be in control of our will, that too is our right and we are working on our own individual lesson of the Soul.

Spirit is Energy, We are Energy

Awareness of capability makes the life's Earth incarnation an exciting event in Soul evolution. Awareness and understanding free us from the resistance to change and growth. They allow us to seek change, to welcome challenge, to live with the love and freedom of life. They allow us to choose the path of growth, without fear of recrimination, judgment, and loss. There is no loss in life, there is only change. What has been will always be. We have been part of Spirit, we are part of Spirit, and we will always be part of Spirit. We cannot be separated from Spirit. Spirit is energy, and we are energy.

Addiction of any type is imprisonment. It locks us into a concept, a person, a thought, a food, a drug, a chemical and it takes away that freedom that allows for growth and change in all human beings. It is destructive to our physical body, our mind, our Soul, and our Spirit. Controlling addiction must start with an awareness that the addiction exists. Becoming aware of an addiction requires that we acknowledge that addiction to ourselves and to anyone else that has agreed to guide us in the removal of the addiction.

Acknowledgement is the first fear to overcome. Next we must have the intention of release. We must give up our addiction. If you are an addict, seek help. There are serious drug addictions in our world that are accepted by people as normal. They will remain problems until the addiction is acknowledged not only by the individuals but by our society. The first reality in overcoming addiction is to restore the physical self to the balance of Nature. This reduces the stress of the physical and the mental. Loving support and the persistence of time will be the other necessary elements for removing our attachment.

Many Souls on Earth feel that they have an addiction to food. Indeed, they do. Others have an addiction to eating. Here, too, we must strive to preserve the balance within the physical. The change needs to be in the quality of food, as well as the quantity. The quality of Nature's food will offer balance, which will relieve the mind and body's craving. Addictions such as foods, eating, and sexual activities should be approached in the same way that all addictions are approached. The results of any addiction can be destructive to our lifestyle and our life, if they are continued. When we find ourselves stuck in life, we can choose to create disease to abort life.

Be Honest

Look at your life with discernment. Are you bored? Are you lonely? Are you fat? Are you too thin? Do you need a different sex partner every night? Do you discriminate in your choice of sex partners? Are you happy? Do you spend time socializing with your friends? Do you spend time with your inner self? Do you spend time being nice to yourself? These are some questions you can ask yourself. Do not fear the answers. Be honest in your discernment.

If your life is not working for you, change it. Find what you desire in life to make you happy. Create a new lifestyle. Do not be afraid. Send love to others with your thoughts and they will come back to you double in size and bursting with light. Involve yourself in activities. Socialize with your friends. Spend time caring about you. Spend thirty minutes each day in meditation. Speak to the guides that are around you and ready to help you. Love those who love you. They are your life line to change. Awareness of addiction, acknowledgement of addiction and learning to dissolve attachment to addiction will give you the time and energy to know the joy of health.

KATHY ODDENINO

HEALING

LESSONS IN WILL, INTENT, AND HEALING

Healing has many meanings. In our world it is a word that is used primarily to describe an external process, where one person makes another person well. This is not a true perspective. Healing, as we know it, is an illusion. Healing is an internal process, which requires the will and intention to be well. The intent to be healed, and the will to do what is necessary to make that happen, allows healing to occur. Will and intent are our actions, healing is the reaction that occurs within our physical body. In some respects of reality, we are all healers of each other. External healing is more of a catalytic process than an actual healing process. A word, a look, a thought, a book or a peaceful moment can be the catalyst that gives us the understanding of will and intent within the body and mind of self to create their own healing.

At the moment we feel the will and intent to become well, our body starts the healing process. The will and intent to be healed is not the intellectual process of thinking that we want to be well. Healing is the process of knowing that we are well. It is understanding at a Soul level that disease does not serve us anymore. Healing is changing our belief system and it is also healing our thoughts about food, water, and air, which are always the true catalyst of healing.

The body is the temple for the Dual Soul and it resembles any other house when it is in need of repair. *Magic wands do not work.* Healing or restoration of our house may take hours, days, weeks, months or years. We must simply hold our will and intent focused. The time required depends on our understanding and will to succeed. Healing self requires a strong knowing and commitment that we desire health and that we have the will and intention to create health as our focus in life.

Absolutely nothing, whether it is medical, chemical, personal or psychic energy, can heal a Soul that does not wish to be healed. When miracle healings occur it is because the will and intent are already focused. The psychic energy gives the process an energy boost and the focus is completed. We have the power with a well-focused will and intent, to heal ourselves very quickly. The healing will seem to be complete, despite the fact that further restoration will continue to occur within our physical and emotional self. This is as it must be. The healing that we know and experience is a healing of the mind as well as our physical body.

When we understand the healing benefits of love, caring, positive communications and support, we will truly understand our role as healers. The energy of love makes each of us a miracle healer. When we relate to people in a giving, caring way, we are sending them the energy of healing. If they have the will and intent to be well, we will renew their energy and give them the strength they need to start the healing process. This approach to healing is more powerful than all the drugs and machines we have created. Much of the caring in our medical community has been lost because of the lack of time. It is difficult to care about someone that you do not know, and that you do not have the time to communicate with freely on a caring basis. Medicine today replaces caring with machines and prescriptions, but in our space and time it is more costly to our lives and less healing is truly accomplished.

We are searching for love. We are searching for identity. We are searching for validation of self. Validation of self cannot be dispensed in a bottle or taken from a machine. The time that a healer spends in sending a patient love by caring, by listening, and by communicating renews the energy forces of the physical body more rapidly and completely than any other method of treatment. This transference of love energy is our world's most valuable medicine. Many good things result from this overall process that impact on both the patient and healer. There is a change in the awareness level of all Souls involved, which is the direct reaction of the energy exchange. The subconscious recognizes and acknowledges the energy of will and intent, as well as the energy of the lesson that is learned. One true healing can change all of Earth's vibrations for us.

As Earth Souls, we are limited by our belief system. Our belief system says we will die if, if, if. The fear of death develops pure panic in our minds. This panic about the fear of death creates the illusion of disease, before disease is physically present. The basis of all fear is the fear of separation. The fear of death becomes the illusion the mind creates, with the image of separation from the physical body. We do not yet understand that there is no death. The Spirit is inexhaustible. We are Spirit. The body is physical matter. All physical matter returns to dust as the energy of life leaves the body.

The care that we give our physical body determines the length of time it will serve us in this existence. When the house of our Spirit is neglected, it may be necessary to leave this life incarnation before all lessons have been learned. All Earth incarnations require a physical body. There is no other way. Learning to look at and treat our physical body with love and to understand the lessons that it wants us to learn is the act of healing ourselves.

All disease, accidents, and trauma are lessons for the Soul. Understand that no one dies until we have made the decision to leave Earth. Acceptance of this reality gives us an understanding of the Soul's control of our own reality and our own world. We come to Earth for Soul evolution. Soul evolution is the learning of lessons that can only occur in physical form. These are not the only lessons that a Soul must learn, but Earth was created as a school for Soul evolution and life is the classroom. Earth incarnations are essential to Soul growth.

Knowing that death is not an end but rather a new beginning allows us to view physical death in more loving terms. When a Soul finds itself in a position of purely human awareness, where Soul awareness is restricted, we will know that it may no longer be possible to learn Soul lessons. We may, with this Soul understanding, choose death as our healing. This too is an Earth lesson and allows death to become a true part of healing. The choice is always that of the Soul.

We do not incarnate on Earth for eternal physical life. Only the Spirit is eternal. Conscious control of life and death are our Earth goals. This is a combination of lessons in Will, Intent, and Healing. All lessons are an effort to maximize the positive sources of energy, within the Universal consciousness. In human terms we can easily visualize the maximization of positive energy, by understanding the balance we are seeking between the body, mind and Spirit. This is our attempt to equalize the love (Spirit), fear (mind) and the physical (body). This is the basis of each of our lessons in our human form. *Learning is, in all respects, healing.*

The fear of dying and death is at this point an obsession. It is the result of a mechanistic, scientific, religious culture that has taught us to believe in everything except ourselves and our eternal energies. A machine cannot keep the Spirit alive. The Spirit is life. It is freedom. We can keep the physical matter of the body alive for long periods, but for what purpose? Is this to protect us from our guilt? Is it to encourage our ego? If the Soul chooses to leave, preserving the physical matter is not in keeping with life. There is no life without the Spirit. There is no death in terms of the Spirit. The Spirit is eternal energy and will always live. That which is Spirit cannot die. There is no opposite of living. Death is an illusion.

Our Spiritual Prospectus is Designed with Great Care

A Soul consciously travels in the higher realms of the Universe during life and at the time of death. The transition of death in physical terms is a "coming home" for the Soul. Living as a Spirit is a deserved rest from the frantic pace of human existence. Spirit life is a time of evaluation and planning. It is a time of peace. It is a time of reuniting with friends. Spirit life is the Universal healing.

The next life incarnation is planned for carefully with guides and participants. Those Souls that may be in human form are contacted and their participation planned. The Spiritual prospectus is designed with great care. All of the goals and lessons are created and understood. This can take any length of time in our concept of time. In the Universal concept time IS. It is one with All That Is.

Healing is by Universal law an individual responsibility.

It is appropriate to seek guidance in the process of healing, because this accelerates learning. We all need teachers and guides. It is a Universal design that we have adopted as an image of the Spirit World. The interaction of Souls allows the teacher to be the pupil, and the pupil to be the teacher. That which is given is returned twofold. Earth today has become a world of placing responsibility and blame, rather than a world of accepting responsibility for self. Failure to accept responsibility has created an imbalance that teaches the lesson of balance. Balance is a lesson for the masses as well as the individual. Accepting responsibility is a creation of balance. In the past cultures of Earth, failure to accept responsibility, which is the result of resistance to intellectual evolution, has led to destruction. Destruction need not be if we are willing to heal and be healed at the Universal level.

Healing is an internal process.

We can practice healing in a very practical manner. On a Soul level and on a cellular level healing the physical is very clearly understood. It is our mind that sets up intellectual and ego energy blocks to our own healing. The Earth process of healing is having the Spiritual Will and Intent to be well, coordinated with the mind intent and will to make this happen. We must then provide the physical elements necessary for physical restoration. *This body-mind and Spirit-mind coordination must be accepted with the*

Joy and Happiness of knowing health. We must be the Joy of Health.

The Joy of Health is the total energy balance of the body, mind and Spirit. This is a total process of balancing the self that will heal, if the Soul truly wants to be healed. If the Soul does not wish to be healed, we do not have the Spiritual Will and Intent to be well. We are involved in another lesson. Healing is not our Soul focus.

Healing abides by the Universal Law of Action and Reaction. We cannot produce the reaction of healing without the balancing actions of body, mind and Spirit that are necessary. This is why healing is an internal process. The attachment of illusion is the major impediment to healing. Illusion is a false belief. The belief in something that is not true will hold us in the negative energy of dis-ease and disease. True disease is a reaction to our actions that will provide a lesson for Soul evolution.

Any action that destroys our positive energy balance as physical humans will result in a negative energy reaction within our physical body, which will enhance the diseases of the mind, body, and Spirit energy. Negative energy is manifested in physical matter as disease. There are no accidents in health or disease, just as there are no accidents in other aspects of our life. We are never a victim. We are creators. We are equal participants in this drama of life. Awareness of that participation and the meaning that it holds for us on Earth will add to the energy vibrations of the Earth itself in a very positive and healing manner. We did not come to Earth only to learn to heal ourselves. The energy that we are is committed to healing the Earth and the Universe too, because they are one with us.

Awareness allows us to care about ourselves and others equally. It recognizes the Spirit self of each and every Soul on Earth. It allows true Soul growth, physical growth, and intellectual growth. It encourages us to BE. This is the Law of Action and Reaction. All Universal Laws are Laws of Creation. They cannot be changed. The Law of Action and Reaction is important in the world of health and healing. Each and every action produces a reaction. The reaction can occur on a mental level, physical level, or Spiritual level. But for reaction to occur, the mind must initiate the action. The direct reaction will always impact on the balance of the trilocular self.

The trilocular design of self, which is integrated balanced energy, can never function without the influence of the energy of all component parts. This assures us that all action will be integrated action. We are all inherently integrated, but we differ in the degree of integration in adult life. Integration is a decrease in singular living by some Souls as they convert to a commonality of living energy within the same level. The trilocular design of self is duplicated throughout our energy system. The mind that serves as the bridge to the Spirit and body is of Spirit and body. The mind is within itself trilocular. The mind is rational, intellectual and intuitive. The mind is body, mind and Spirit within itself, which is essentially three types of energy within itself.

All of self is designed from energy, in the nesting concept of energy within energy within energy. Each source of energy is a trilocular unit that repeats itself throughout the energy of self and throughout Earth and the Universe. The action of any part of self sets up a reaction of vibratory response within all parts of self. An example of this is the action of physical activity. As we grow chronologically, our mind, operating from its belief system, says we are aging and therefore should become less active. We respond to this belief by decreasing our activity level and accepting the concept of "old age." Age is of the mind, not the body. The concept of age is accompanied by the concept of physical deterioration. The unspoken message to the physical body is "I don't need you anymore." This message allows the reaction of "shut down" to occur in the physical sense.

The body starts to decrease absorption of calcium as it decreases activity. Other nutrients become less important. Eating becomes less important. The physical self goes into hibernation. The mind is telling it to deteriorate and the body is coordinating the reaction. The action of the mind produces the reaction within the body. Deterioration is common when a Soul retires from a career focus. Many people believe that retirement is a period of non-productivity. If the belief also is such that retirement means we are through with life, then death will occur soon after the event of retirement. Retirement gives us the perfect opportunity to do the things that we have always wanted to do but have not had enough time to do them.

The action occurs within the mind and the body experiences the reaction, each and every time that our body is compromised. The action within the thinking mind is rational, intellectual, and intuitive. The ego focus of the mind expands our negative mind. The integrated action of the mind becomes an integrated reaction of the body, mind, and Spirit. All mind concepts relating to age, retirement, physical deterioration and death are illusions of our belief system. We can heal ourselves of all these actions and reactions by changing our belief system. The same concept holds true with disease. If our father died of a heart attack at the age of 40, and we hold the belief that because of a genetic link the same death will happen to us, it will. The mind is the builder, the body is the result. We can also look at "the father's death" as an opportunity to understand our own health better, and to live longer.

This is the mind-body coordination that is not recognized totally within our world. Dis-ease or disease is a product of the mind first. The body supports the concept. It is the concept of the mind that says "all food is good food" that allows us to eat to our physical deterioration. The integration of action and reaction within the body, mind, and Spirit is so sensitively interrelated that it is difficult in physical human terms to visualize where one begins and the other ends. We cannot totally understand this relationship until we have gained in total understanding. We must exercise faith and trust in the knowing to open our mind to the awareness, which will lead to the understanding and integration of our life circumstances. This concept of action and reaction is hard for us to imagine, as it occurs within the cellular levels of our body. The words to explain it in human understanding are not used because this concept is not understood by the level of today's mind. For a concept that will help the imagination let me use another example. This illustration will show you the vibratory energy force of self.

You have a calm lake of water at your feet. You pick up a pebble from the shore and you drop it from the level of your head into the water. Watch the vibratory response of the water. See the circles of energy spread wider and wider into the stillness of the water? The energy force of the pebble, and the energy force with which the pebble fell, created the action that caused the energy vibratory reaction within the water. There were several layers of action and reaction that occurred before the pebble hit the water. In your mind a thought occurred first. You picked up the pebble, as a reaction to the thought. You lifted the pebble to the level of your head, secondary to a thought. You dropped the pebble as a reaction to another thought. Each of these energy forces occurred one within the other as connected energy.

This same "nesting" concept of energy creates our world. It is at once integrated and separate. It is the act of creation and it is the creation. We create our own reality. When this is understood, the Soul progress will be much more rapid and can effect healing instantly in the thought process. The power for healing increases with the conscious practice of energy control. Healing will happen by degrees for many Souls, depending upon the current level of progress. The will and intent to understand healing and to have this creation as part of our life, will allow it to BE. It will start the vibratory response of the positive energy force in motion, which will increase with each vibration to help us heal ourselves.

The healing professions will revert to love and relating as a primary therapy for future medical practice. Touching, communicating, caring, and sharing are all healing forms. They are positive energy forces that set the pattern of vibratory response within the patient. Allowing these forms to be practiced openly, and accepting their practice personally, will be healing itself for the medical world. We will be dropping a pebble in the water and we will see the energy expand and grow. This will be teaching healing to the masses. The teachers for this healing evolution are now on Earth. It will BE. Today's healers will soon understand their expanded role as teachers of love on Earth. There is much to be done in this energy force to help us to understand ourselves.

At this moment on Earth, medical science has reached the level of tremendous scientific knowledge. This is the moment in our evolution to bridge the gap between self-healing of the total person and scientific healing which will allow us the freedom to re-evaluate our personal creations in life. There is at present a critical imbalance created by our primary focus being on the scientific. Science can jeopardize life when it is out of balance. It can jeopardize the entire system that is being created, when it fails to maintain the balance. To treat dis-ease from a scientific basis is compounding the problem, not healing the problem.

A new evaluation of the true meaning of life is in progress upon Earth. The energy vibrations that are being generated will be felt by all of humankind. This new meaning of life will occur because of our need to understand ourselves. It will be a Spiritual awakening that will allow us to be a balanced trilocular being that is whole and free in positive energy. It will be an individualized healing that will effect a planetary healing. Healers are the Earth's catalyst for the transference of healing energy. They can polarize the power of that energy, and teach the concept of using that internal energy to everyone. Within us is the cure for all of our diseases.

The knowledge of the elements of the Earth, the mind, and the heart are the sources of our healing energy. This energy must work together to be a total healing force. When our belief system accepts this Universal reality, then it will be. The rhythm of the Earth and the rhythm of man will be in unison and there will be a new awareness. We can combine the healing methods of today with the Universal healing methods in a very practical and effective manner. The process must start within the home. Corporate big business is our most derogatory energy to affect human health and longevity.

Changing our eating practices will start us on the perfect path to health. Our society has ventured far from the concept of Nature's food. Our world is one of processed food and fast food that has been virtually stripped of the Earth elements that we need for our internal chemical balance. What we have in fast food is the exact opposite of what the body truly needs. We have a food intake that is based on fat, sugar, starch, salt and chemicals. This leaves our cells starved for the elements of Nature. We suffer cravings, longings, searchings and disease. Our food puts us out of balance with the chemical, physical creation that we are designed to be.

Spirit designed us, in its own image, as an integrated unit. When the body is out of balance, the mind and Spirit are out of balance and disease is created. Disease is our creation of our personal reality. We live in a Universe that abides by the Law of Cause and Effect and the Law of Action and Reaction. We will always react to our actions. Our society's food does not create cellular vibrations of pure positive energy. Our energy vibratory response is that of dropping a feather into the clear pool of water. Nothing happens. There is no energy generated within the electrical energy system of the cellular structure. It creates energy that is negative energy of desperation, of searching, of craving, and of fear for the survival of self.

Most acts of violence in our society are created by people who fail to maintain the positive cellular energy within their body, which allows them to respond in fear. This imbalance is created by the wrong foods, drugs, chemicals, and a dramatic fear focus. The fear for survival generates negative energy that impacts upon our entire society. This is a creation of imbalance of body, mind and Spirit. We can be healed from within by changing the action without. We can choose to drop a pebble into the water of life instead of dropping a feather.

Changing the belief system of our human population is the first step to healing ourselves. Changing our behaviors and actions is the second step to healing ourselves. Learn to seek relaxation through exercise, Neural Depolarization, playing, dancing and swimming – the fun things of childhood that bring joy to your heart. Use simple excursions into exploring your life that are fun, spontaneous, and free. Share your home with someone you love. Encourage the relationships of families and friends to become closer and more supportive of individual and group living. Generate love to light the heart and Soul of everyone you meet. Share thoughts, feelings and emotions from a core level. Communication improves appreciation for each other, and builds the respect that gives one the freedom to love totally.

Lessons will always be there for each of us to learn. Our lessons will make disease and trauma part of our world, but the healing can be true learning for our Soul. Seek medical care with the desire to learn what our lesson may be. Only we will know, but our healers can be our guides and our teachers in the exploration and healing. As we open our thinking mind, the solution to all challenges will be easier to see as healing. Use scientific medical capabilities to repair and support. We must not refuse to accept the responsibility for the final creation. It is our creation and without the acknowledgement of the lesson, our healing is not complete. Acknowledge the lesson and release it. The positive energy of support will send us healing from within.

Healing is a creation of personal reality. It is within each of us. Listen to the energy vibrations of your feeling-tone. We can control our own healing, with the will and intent to live in health. *Healing becomes a practical exercise of focusing the mind on the joy of health.* Knowing that we are free of disease is a joyous experience. Focusing the mind on health requires active changes in our belief system and lifestyle to support our mind in an understanding of health. Total unity of self is required in healing self. Knowing that we create disease through fear and faulty support of the physical chemical system will allow a new creation of health and happiness.

Disease is the reaction to inappropriate action. Health is the reaction to appropriate action. When this becomes the understanding and the focus of our mind, the Spirit will react with joy and happiness to accept a body in vibrant health. The body will react to this new mind focus by restoration, rejuvenation, and positive energy. We will find peace in the joy of health.

LOVE

Each emotion, each feeling, all of reality has an opposite. The opposite of love is fear. For those of you who mentally jumped to hate – hate is fear and therefore also the opposite of love. The English language allows these duplicities which can sometimes be confusing. Love, as a concept, is not acceptable to most men. Many men feel foolish even thinking the word, never mind saying it out loud. Love translates into sex in most men's minds. These dear Souls are truly the uninitiated. Love is equal to mother's milk! It is truly the nectar of the Spirits and it is the strongest emotion in the human mind.

The fear of commitment keeps us from understanding love. We envision commitment as loss of freedom. Dwell on this for a moment internally, to grasp the awareness of how opposites truly work. If we fear our loss of freedom with love, we will always live with resistance to both love and commitment. Love is not only giving love, but love is also being open to receiving love. Giving and receiving love can both create the fear of the loss of freedom. When we live without the benefit of love in our life, we live in fear. This fear of love is a learned belief in our society and it can easily be translated as a fear of commitment.

When we don't understand the emotion of love, it is our attachment to the opposite energy as physical sex that prevents us from understanding love. When we cannot understand love and are not aware that there is an opposite of our belief, we are showing ourselves exactly where we are in the design of our Dual Soul and its level of evolution. This is the ideal way to evaluate our own progress with Soul evolution. Love encompasses a multitude of emotions and feelings, but sex is a physical act. The lesser emotions are offshoots of the primary emotions and have lesser capacity to function as an overall concept. Some of our normal emotions are gladness, happiness, joy, enchantment, ecstasy, beatitude, and many, many others. All are essentially expressions of love.

Love can cause a rush of blood through our body that suddenly makes us feel like we are enveloped in a warm, fuzzy cocoon. It is peaceful, sweet, loving, and joyful. It is health. It is the shining white light of Spiritual protection. Love dilates our blood vessels and carries vital oxygen to each and every cell in our body. It helps us grow as an energy of body, mind, and Spirit. Love broadens our concept of humanity. It makes friends out of enemies. It opens our heart and allows our Spirit to bloom as a rose blooms in the spring. It makes work play. It gives the mind the freedom to soar. Love is life, it is Spirit, and it is hope. It truly is the nectar of the Spirit.

Love is the appreciation of and joining of love that enhances the evolution of the Soul. Love's reality is the Spirit of the body and brain. Without love we have no Spirit, no hope, and no joy for the living. We have severe damage to one of our integrated parts. The Spirit – the infinite energy - the Spirit part of us, is also the happy, joyful loving part of us. It is the emotional, feeling part of our humanity. All death is conceptually destruction of the Spirit's true essence in matter. The integration of the Spirit is absolute. Without the energy of the Spirit, the mind and the physical body will be on a self-destructive course until they acknowledge the Spirit's freedom to BE. This will not be a conscious path of self-destruction, but rather it will be a conscious, frantic, and endless search for identity and self-recognition within the physical world.

The Spirit, although sharing equal billing while in human form, is the eternal energy of us that never dies. The Spirit is our eternal life. The Spirit is the "Spirit self" in all humans. The Spirit is the core of us. The Spirit is the eternal love of man. The Spirit is the part of us that is consciously working towards the perfection of the energy of our Soul evolution. The Soul is the part of us that struggles to develop inner peace, understanding and forgiveness. It is the part of us that tries to learn to be non-judgmental in the face of hostility and untruth. This is the part of us that holds truth in total reverence, seeing the purity and promise of living Spirit energy in action and the beauty in the essence of fulfillment. Our Spirit is honesty, trust, gentleness, tolerance, joy, defenselessness, patience, faithfulness, open-mindedness, generosity, hope and love. To honor our internal Spirit energy is to honor the true self as energy.

To commit to the true essence of the Spirit is to commit to the internal Spirit Energy. That commitment becomes the shining light of love. The opposite of love is fear. Fear is not the devil's doing. The only devil in our Universe is us. In our devil disguise, we can indeed wreak havoc with our Spirit Consciousness through our denial. The disease of our Spirit inactiveness is primarily self-directed, because of our failure to understand the true process of our Soul Evolution which expands our Spirit Consciousness. Understanding that the Spirit of us is an eternal energy, therefore, life for us is eternal, removes our fear of separation that we have captured and cling to tightly as our fear concept of death.

When we can view death as a new beginning and not an ending, we will no longer fear the separation that we are dramatically afraid will happen. Once death is understood, the cause for resistance ceases to be. The need to "fight for life," whether done figuratively or literally, ceases to be important because love is a living energy and the Spirit is eternal. At the moment of death, we begin to see ourselves as the Spirit creatures that we truly are. We see the worth, the talent, the contribution that we are capable of giving to the Universal Energy and we can at last stop our criticism of ourselves and our life.

When we stop judging ourselves we stop judging other people. When we start loving ourselves, we start loving other people. We begin to realize that we are perfect just the way that we are. We start searching for the lesson to be found in where we are. We find ourselves excited about the next step forward. We rejoice in our humanity and find sharing a Spiritual blessing. We suddenly realize that each of us has a Spirit, even if it is sleeping, and we begin to accept the challenge of teasing it to wakefulness. Denial of our true Spirit means we must live life over and over again and again until we finally learn how to love each other.

Remember the first time you rode a bicycle? You wobbled back and forth, ran into the gate, bumped your toe so hard you broke it and then you flew over the handlebars and skidded in the gravel on your face. This happened to me. I grew up without learning to ride a bicycle. When I was in my twenties I decided to learn. Unfortunately, I tried to learn on a large downhill grade. I lost control of the bicycle and abused my body in the fall. I hit my head on a pole and lost consciousness for a few moments. I learned to ride the bicycle, but I totally lost my passion for riding. Life is like trying to ride a bicycle sometimes. Not all paths are smooth. But you get up, despite the hardness of the fall, and get back on that bicycle you learned to ride through the various challenges of life. You may indeed fall again and again as you attempt to learn and grow, but bruises are memories of the physical self and the mind trying to reach attunement with the Spirit. Our bruises should be cherished, kissed and cared for, not cried over.

When our heart starts to bloom with love, fear will be the first bee to fly away. Love and fear are not compatible to live in the same house so they will never dwell together in the same heart for very long. As opposites, the positive energy flow will cancel the negative energy flow if the heart is allowed to grow. If we find ourselves operating from a basis of fear we are presenting dark energy to our body, mind and Spirit. The dark energy contracts the blood vessels, constricts the lungs, squeezes the cells until they are starved for oxygen and an energy block will form. This dark energy begins to multiply within itself until dis-ease becomes a reality for the body, mind, and Spirit to live with. Dis-ease always escalates to disease unless the negative flow of energy can be interrupted and overcome with positive energy.

Fear is a disease of the mind, which will soon manifest itself as a disease of the Soul and physical body because it has begun to affect the cellular pattern within the body. The vibrational pattern of the positive energy flow of the cellular structure has been blocked. There is no disease known that cannot be healed if the body, mind, and Spirit choose to actively engage in restructuring the cellular energy patterns. Once the mind frees itself of fear, anger, hate, dishonesty, guilt, sin and despair it can confront the issue of healing in total love.

An absolute release of negative energy must be accomplished before healing is permanent. Each negative energy force of life does not have to be dealt with as a separate force. The negative energy force within the self is a failure to love. This love can be directed as a total energy force of forgiveness of self and others. Forgiveness is love. When the Spirit, Dual Soul and physical body are free, they can form the union for healing the body with love. Healing then constitutes an entire re-patterning of the cellular structure that formulates the disease process. Complete healing will include an overall cellular restructuring to assure permanency. Healing is love. Love is healing.

A Soul that has truly decided to leave Earth will not be healed because the Spirit and the Soul will not agree to work in unison with the conscious mind. It is still beneficial to the evolution of the Soul to free the Soul and Spirit of fear and its tributary emotions. Releasing fear is a challenge of many incarnations for some Souls. If we can learn it well, we may never have to learn it again. If it isn't comfortable for us, we will accept it as a challenge in another life and we may or may not start again at the beginning, depending upon our awareness level in the thinking mind.

The Spirit is the infinite part of the human body. Our Spirit is manifested in our heart. Our Spirit works in unison with our Dual Soul. The Spirit contains the "best of the human" which is chosen from our Soul experience. Our Spirit Consciousness is the Spirit within us that lives from the pattern of the Ethical Values that is the energy part of our human design. Our Soul can be most clearly identified as our subconscious mind. The Soul is our energy aura that is evolving in the physical reality of life. It is the energy of all human memory of the Soul experiences of the human being.

Some of us may have our Soul memories so deeply covered over that we have only a tiny aura. This small film may be a dismal, dull grey, brown, or black. This is truly a depressed Soul. The Soul that has love shining in its aura will appear as a beautiful rainbow. The colors will pulsate and change in intensity and quantity as the thoughts and emotions change in the thinking mind. At times some energy will be predominant or perhaps missing, which depends on the physical behavior that is being lived.

Everything experienced by our Spirit is reflected in our mind and body. Have you heard it said of a kind and loving man, that he has a big heart or a big Spirit? Have you heard it said of a selfish, fearful man, that he has no Spirit at all? What we do is a good indication of who we are, in that precise moment in time. The truth is a reflection of the actions which result from our thoughts, and the more each person lives his or her Ethical Values, the more the Spirit Energy can be seen as it protects the body. Truth may not be reflected in our words if we have not consciously learned to live our Ethical Values. If we have a well-developed Spirit, it will be apparent in our daily life, because our Ethical Values will be reflected in our physical behavior. We will be the living essence of our Spirit Energy.

True Emotional Health of the mind is Spiritual Growth.

Each of the parts has its own roles to play but no individual part escapes the influence of the other two. If the Spirit can be true to its Spirit image, the mind and body will be healthier and constantly sharing in the growth of the Soul. This sharing allows for the development of more awareness within the mind and body through the motivation of love. This awareness affects the development of the rational mind, the intellectual mind, the intuitive mind and the physical body. True emotional health of the mind is Spiritual growth. No one can be living true emotional health without living the Ethical Values that are the design of our Spirit Energy.

We must go back to our example of the mother bearing twins - if mother is healthy then they all should be healthy, but if she isn't then they are all at the same risk. Our body, mind and Spirit work from the same level of integration. In today's society it is difficult to give the Spirit its true freedom. Our cultural beliefs have made the mind the controller. Not only do we rely upon the intellectual mind to the extreme, but our reliance is focused on the ego mind force that has no Ethical Values to guide it.

The intellectual mind is not capable of feeling without using the Spirit energy. The intellectual mind gathers and stores data. It is capable of absorbing information and regurgitating information. This is not true learning. True learning is intelligence. It is information that is assimilated, perceived and acted upon with "feeling" in relationship to the circumstance. There must be a combination of rational and intuitive thinking that accompanies the intellectual mind. If all three mind forces were not essential to the thinking process Spirit would not have given them to us. When we can think with love and caring as part of consciousness, the energy of the Ethical Values is easier to absorb and use.

Our body is not designed with unusable excesses. Everything has its purpose. To be whole we must be aware of, appreciate, and utilize each and every sense or capability that we possess. The mind that we consciously use, the intellectual mind, depends upon the five senses being acute. We accept these five senses. Many people today still deny that we have other senses available for use. Our Human design has many senses that we do not use. Every person has identical capabilities. This book is an indication of the use of another of those senses. The many incarnations that Souls have experienced have provided the Soul with unlimited "knowing." The knowing is there to be used when the mind is ready to open to the using. When we understand the love of self, we will be able to know the power of our total existence as both matter and energy, which allows us to get more out of our physical lives.

Human civilization, at this time in history, has the potential to become a superhuman race by using the power of Universal Intelligence. Using the three forces of the mind freely will allow rapid evolution on Earth. If Earth progress is guided by the Spirit, Soul evolution will move rapidly into the area of perfection. The primary goal of using Earth as a school has always been to perfect the evolution of the Dual Soul. Evolution of the Dual Soul is understanding love and living the Ethical Values. Earth is a plane of Spirit Consciousness that is teaching each and every person about life and love.

Earth is a level of Spiritual existence in physical form. On Earth other Spiritual planes exist that are inhabited by Souls who are resting from Earth's physical plane. Incarnations can manifest into countless returns to the physical plane of Earth before any individual Soul reaches the point where they can pass into a non-physical plane. Souls on other Earth planes have the role of guides and teachers. These are lower levels of the Spiritual plane where the Souls are involved in teaching the lesson of love to those on the physical plane. They are caretakers, guardian angels of the physical Souls on Earth.

Love is a concept that can only be understood in stages of learning. The higher the level of the Soul the higher the level of pure shining Love. The slow development of Soul evolution on Earth is primarily due to the physical belief system that locks our focus into the development of the intellect. Intellect in itself is a matter of perception of importance. Our intellectual focus may be different, but no one focus is less important than the other. The difference occurs in the type of data collected by the Dual Soul.

Belief systems have always controlled cultures. Cultures have varied in beliefs and do change through the centuries, but basically they remain archaic compared to the Spirit world. Beliefs limit us. Living a belief is equivalent to attaching chains to one's head, throat, arms, waist and ankles. If we think other than what people expect us to think, we won't be accepted. If we speak of anything other than what coincides with current beliefs, no one will listen. If we build something other than what regulations allow, they will make us tear it down. If we eat something that isn't what is currently advertised, we are strange. If we choose to be where others aren't, we don't know how to get along with people. All of our human assumptions are simply assumptions, not truth.

We are afraid to live without adhering to the beliefs of society because we are afraid that if we do we will not be loved. We believe that "conformity assures love." This is a belief of our culture that has captured young minds and created countless problems within our society. To drop all beliefs and just be would do much for our world. People are perfect just the way Spirit made them. We don't have to be life-long subscribers to an outdated belief system. It is the failure to be all that Spirit made us that allows us to be imperfect in the physical realm. It is okay to use all of our Spirit-given senses, not just five of them.

Belief systems drain tremendous amounts of creative energy from the human form through their fettering systems. This drained energy is a dark energy as another blocking of energy that takes its needs out on the physical body. The blocking of energy by our beliefs is the cause of many diseases in our society. If a Soul can find no way to release this energy block, it will choose death to abort the life design. The Soul will manifest dying in its own fashion to make its own statement. With death the Soul has chosen a way out of the restriction and will try again with a different set of circumstances. Because death is many times the only escape that a Soul can see from its human state, it will make that choice as its alternative. Choosing death as an escape before the completion of the lesson results in many, many incarnations passing before one lesson can be completed.

Belief systems essentially control us. They control our relationship to Spirit, our mind and our body. If we are taught one specific religious belief, we may not change it for a lifetime or many lifetimes. To do so, in our belief, would send us to hell and the fires of damnation. This is an illusion we have created. Spirit's joy is in seeing the growth of Her children. We can love Spirit simply by loving the Spirit in us. We can also accept that there is a Supreme Being and love Spirit with no other conditions being necessary. Spirit is simply a higher and more advanced form of energy than our human lives today.

The true Spirit is such that if we truly love ourselves, we love the Spirit within us. Many people think they love themselves but they are frequently paying homage to their ego instead. Loving yourself gives you the freedom to love all. Loving yourself is the supreme test of the internal struggle between the ego who wants to control and the Spirit self who wants to be free and loving. Freedom to love all does not refer to the sexual freedom to love all, which has been our physical interpretation. Loving all in sexual freedom is the opposite of the Spiritual freedom of loving all. Sexual freedom is, in effect, total control by the physical body. Exploitation of sexual freedom is one of the most confining controls we know. It is a disease of our body, mind, Spirit and Soul. It is the opposite of love in marriage. It is a fear of solitude.

Our belief system therefore affects our Spirit and how it is allowed to be. It affects the love we are able to give and the love that we are able to receive. It affects our ego and the value systems we adopt as our gauges for living. It affects our intellect and the information we gather. It affects our senses and the freedom we give them. It affects the life that we live and the person that we are. It affects the relationships of our world. It affects the attachments of our life.

Beliefs also affect the ultimate growth of the physical body, through the mind. The body's cellular patterning is strongly influenced and controlled by the belief system. When we believe something about our body, it will immediately set to work to make that belief come true. The body is like a puppet on the string of the mind and Spirit. It is literally built by our thoughts, beliefs, attitudes and needs. The body is made sick or well by what we believe it to be.

The mind is the builder, the body is the result. No one ever develops a disease unless he does it to himself. We create our own physical reality. Yet there is no disease known that cannot be healed if the mind and Spirit choose to heal it. The body, mind and Spirit together can rebuild, restore, regenerate, and rejuvenate the body totally. None of this will happen without an understanding and acceptance of love which will pattern our physical behaviors through the Ethical Values.

The body is constantly changing, but our images do not change because we have strong beliefs about how we look, what we think and how we feel. To change the appearance of the body it is necessary to first change our belief in the image of self. The image that we cling to is the ego's identity image. There is great strength in being able to change the image of self. It is an act of the Spirit in controlling the ego.

Most disease is the direct result of an energy block. This energy block may be in any part of the integrated whole. If we have an energy block, a disease, we must work on all parts of the whole to create a cure. Since the body, mind and Spirit are so tightly entwined, working on one affects all three. Identify your problem and first heal the part that is most closely associated with the disease, but stay open to the other areas with loving influence. Love is the healing Spirit. Love heals our body, mind, Soul and Spirit.

The body is our physical grounding source on Earth. There are many Ethereal Spirits on Earth but we can't see them. They no longer function by our system of conditions and beliefs. You, too, have probably spent some time on Earth in the Spirit form, but for now you have chosen to be human. *The first rule of being human is having a physical body.* Our physical body gives us the right of participation in Earth life. Without it we would be simply another Spirit that no one can see. We have chosen this incarnation to learn. Learning requires participation in the act of life. Learning requires love.

The need for love is understood by our Soul Consciousness at the moment of birth. Our lessons are understood at that time. We have chosen to act out this role of life with other willing participants that have agreed to love us. We begin growth and continue our growth from this basis of love. Everyone knows their lines. But life is like any other stage play. Every now and then someone may ad lib a life and upset the complete dialogue for a couple of centuries, but the Soul purpose is remembered and the play goes on, despite the pause.

As development occurs in human terms the mind is exposed over and over again to the culture, the beliefs, the dogma, the very reality of human existence. All of these exposures are meant to be. They are part of the lesson. They can be a challenge to that belief in, that knowing that we are always loved. *The human challenge is to learn to be a free Spirit, to cope with and to rise above what we experience in the physical world.* The person who lives in fear becomes attached to the emotions and challenges of everyday life. We must choose what we see with our physical eyes and hear with our physical ears. We must exercise free will and we must always think.

Spirit is a higher form of energy than man, and Spirit consistently lives the Ethical Values that we are seeking to learn. Spirit wants us to recognize the value of our Spirit in all of life's physical circumstances because we are infinitely and eternally Spirit Energy. We cannot recognize the Spirit within and not recognize that love is also within. Not only does Spirit want us to recognize the value of our Spirit but we as humans want to recognize the presence of that Spirit. We want to appreciate the Spirit value and learn to trust in it, learn to revere it, to use it, to be it. The Spirit is manifested in many, by the Love of humanity. That is Soul evolution. That is love. In loving the Spirit, we love our internal Spirit self, which gives us the ability to live our Ethical Values as our personality and behavior.

In the beginning, there was light. Spirit is light. When we were still an integrated part of the Spirit energy, we were light. Now we are a child of Spirit and we must learn and appreciate the depth of our being before we can return to light. We were made in the likeness of Spirit. Each Soul developed as a tiny spark of light thrown off from Spirit Source. This is the design of our internal energy source. Some people today are questioning how so many new people arrived on Earth. Spirit in its joyousness throws off more sparks. Spirit in its wisdom creates new thought forms and gives them the opportunity of physical birth. Spirit is happy with the new rhythm of Soul evolution that it sees on Earth. Now Earth has many new Souls as well as many old Souls, and many Souls that are continuing to search for their rhythm and balance.

The old Souls are here to teach a new concept of love. They have gone through Soul evolution and they have tremendous mass energy to assist in this process. New Souls have chosen to be born and other evolving Souls are now coming in even larger numbers to learn the concept of love. Violence and war will soon disappear from the Earth as the Spiritual shift reaches its peak. The Spiritual shift now taking place on Earth is not a religious revolution. This is a Spiritual evolution of Spiritual energy to create the awareness and understanding of love.

Being religious and being Spiritual is not the same thing. Religion, in history, has been a means of controlling the mind, Spirit and physical body. Spiritualism is a movement to understand the self and free the body, mind and Spirit into an awareness of its own energy form. Earth has never had a religion or culture that has not controlled us in some degree, in some way. Spiritualism gives the control to the self through Spirit. Spiritualism is a movement of Love created from within the Spirit World. *Spiritualism is based on the ancient knowledge that was shared by ancient Philosophers and in living the Ethical Values to support a better human and a better Earth.*

Sometimes in today's Spiritual movement it is not easy to get people to gather together. That is because Spiritualism is not a method of control. It is an internal process of learning the history of ourselves as human beings. We do not have to gather together for our energy to connect, but gathering together creates an advanced pull on all energy. It is the energy on the planet that will spread the understanding. It is a personal search for the true self. It is not a search for a leader. Following any leader other than Spirit can be very detrimental to the Dual Soul and Spirit Consciousness.

The physical body, having chosen to be here, is now under the influence of the mind and Spirit. It is our grounding influence, our temple on Earth. What we choose to create in our life and learning depends largely upon our thinking mind, but the result will influence all parts of the integrated whole again. As the number of Spiritual people expands on Earth, Earth will become nicer to us and help with our growth as we become nicer to Earth. Spirit made us as energy beings and put us on Earth. She made us part of the Nature on Earth. She stocked the cupboard of Earth with the foods that will make the body grow. She designed the body and She knows what food works best. She set about making them all part of our natural habitat. She provided for us with the love of caring and sharing.

Spirit didn't make fire, man did. In the beginning, foods were eaten raw. Eating the foods of Nature grounded us even more into our surroundings. Grounding the human body to Earth kept the power of our energy focused in our body where we could use it for survival as we learned to understand our new world. Man as Spirit needs to be grounded to this Earth energy. The grounding of some Spirits is difficult. Some Souls felt restless and unnatural in their new habitat. This prompted us to develop the custom of sharing energy in the form of communities. These communities provided the joining of energies which helped with the grounding process.

This sharing of energy was a subconscious decision in the beginning of life to stabilize the energy and increase the power of learning. Sharing was our subconscious desire to experience the combined energy of love. The family unit was Spirit's original design and has worked very well on Earth. It was designed by Spirit for our benefit, not for "the fall of man," as we have believed. We were designed to have a mate. This design did not happen accidentally. Using this partnership process allowed the Soul to cast itself in the role of either male or female during different incarnations to learn all of the lessons of our physical life. The mating of opposites provided the experience of operating from different focuses at different times. The partnership process also provides the maximum focus of energy and power when the choice is made wisely. This has untold advantages in Soul evolution.

In our world we could compare it to driving a car with an eight-cylinder engine as compared to a car with a four-cylinder engine. The level of power and speed are dramatically different. For a Soul that is focused on its evolution, a Spiritual partnership with a mate of the opposite sex provides that energy boost and allows for total freedom of the Soul in producing children. Love is freedom. A joining of two people of the same sex does not work in the same manner for grounding because of the energy levels. Man and woman have different energy levels designed as the trilocular complements of the Spirit. This provides a more compatible energy balance of the bodies separately, together and in the Universe. The joining of male and female energy completes the energies in the balance Spirit designed. This makes for a smooth flow with the energy points of the body joining together with the energy flows in a smooth and unbroken stream to balance with both individuals in total unity.

In a joining of two energies of the same sex, the energy cords are misshapen, with bulges and spurs protruding from the energy flow. This can cause tremendous energy blocks and tremendous disease processes for the body to deal with. We can see this now in our world. Remember that we can cure all diseases, but healing does require a releasing of those energy blocks. The quality of energy is also recognized by its color and vibrations as well as its texture. Grounding energy is perhaps better known in our world as chakra energy, and as all energy will, it changes depending on the state of our integrated self.

Energy that is presenting an energy block is seen as dark energy or negative, depressive energy. It is visible in shades of grey, brown, and black. A balanced person glows in an array of colors. They flow and change with the joy and love that is being sent and received. An agitated person you could compare to a burning sparkler on the 4th of July. There will be sparks flying off in a shower pattern and they will be shades of red and black. Red in our aura is an indication of strong passion. The type of emotion can be determined by the color of the red. For example, physical passion will be a deep garnet red and anger will be the red of fire.

The interaction of body, mind and Spirit determines our energy flow. If we are in good physical, emotional, and Spiritual health, our energy flow is at its best and will not cause us an energy block or disease. The love that we feel for ourselves, Spirit and our neighbor is the protection we have from disease. The love that we have and the love that we share is our path of Soul growth. Growth is always more complete in the presence of love. Love is Spirit. Love is Earth. Love is Human. Love is Universal.

RELATIONSHIPS

All relationships are Soul lessons. Relationships are essential to Earth life for these lessons and the joy they bring to our Earth experience. Living is joy and happiness. Many Souls must learn to bring this joy and happiness up from their core Soul to enjoy an incarnation. This is one of the lessons of the Dual Soul. The joy and happiness in living is the true reason for living.

No two relationships are the same. This applies to the individual relationships each of us experience and the individual experiences of different people with us. We all live with an energy field. Our energy fields are created from all of our past lives. No two people experience the identical experiences in every lifetime. Relationships are determined basically by the perception of both individuals, and the interaction of these two Souls from their awareness of Soul memories. Soul memories and inner awareness do not at the present time on Earth usually operate from a conscious basis. The perception of a relationship may differ with the individuals involved. The relationship that is perceived with the unity of awareness is the relationship that allows for the most significant growth.

Enlightened Souls will enjoy this awareness, but it is not essential to a casual relationship. Awareness is essential to a meaningful, growth-oriented relationship.

Even without awareness, we will often find ourselves with an immediate like or dislike for individuals that we meet. This emotional reaction is the immediate result of Soul memories or Soul awareness that is operating on a subconscious level. Good relationships contribute to good health and joy. They should be cherished and nourished, just as we would cherish any material possession in our world. A good relationship is far more valuable to our world than any material possession could ever be.

A Soul does not grow without the contact of other Souls. The drama of life would not be much of a drama without the interactions that relationships provide. There are many levels of relationships. There are those we never know even as friends but with whom we have casual contact. There are those we make eye contact with for a brief moment without words or interactions. There are business contacts. There are those whom we call friends that we spend our play time with. There are those we are attracted to as lovers. There are family members. There are those whom we see as kindred Souls that we will marry.

Souls can sometimes recognize each other on a Soul level and want to be near or apart on a conscious level. This happens in all of life, whether or not the consciousness is there. Those with whom we are playing dramas are Souls that we are aware of loving, and with whom we have chosen to play this particular drama.

There is always agreement in relationships on a Soul level. So when we feel inclined to blame the other person for a happening, don't. Always look internally to see what lesson we have designed for ourselves.

The close relationships of family are a good example of our planned experience. Nothing happens by accident. The lessons that we have chosen to learn can be learned best through the relationships that we have planned for our Earth experience. We do not form lasting relationships with everyone that we meet, because they are not coded into our life design for this incarnation. This does not mean that the Soul is unfamiliar to us. Souls frequently incarnate together in cultures and groups as well as in families.

The Soul that we pass on the street, and make casual eye contact with, may leave us with a lasting appreciation of our own worth. This small part was also coded into our drama, and many times it may be a more significant lesson than a relationship that we see as a constant struggle. The reason it is more significant is that for one instant in our space of time we felt joy, love, and appreciation. We may spend our lifetime in some relationships and not have that sense. That tiny flash of true Spiritual recognition and joy can change our entire perception and awareness level of what we are all about and what our life is all about. These Souls are frequently guides who have materialized for that moment of physical encouragement, which they know we desperately need. Accept that joy and hold it within you.

This has happened frequently in my life since childhood. I never understood it until now, but I have remembered each and every guide that has sent me the energy of joy. There have been times in my life when my guides have materialized and spent minutes or hours talking to me. These were times when my physical energy levels were becoming seriously low, and the Spiritual energy of my guides gave my body the extra energy charge that I needed to restore myself. Afterwards I would experience a joy that was seemingly boundless, and I was unable to fully remember how tired I had felt before. Each of these memories has stayed part of my consciousness and has restored me again and again with their collective energy.

Within families there is a constant flow and ebb of familiar energy that brings lessons to the surface, for all to be conscious of and deal with on a daily basis. Those who have chosen to be a part of a large loving family are also saying to the world that they are open and willing to learn. They have chosen a fertile and dramatic playing field as their stage of life. There is less fear to be overcome in this atmosphere of sharing. Those who are learning to overcome fear have asked for multiple supports with their lesson. The other family members involved have lovingly agreed to provide this support. Souls of this caliber do not see only immediate family members as family. They have Soul memories that allow them to gather everyone they meet to themselves as family.

Balancing the body, mind, and Spirit and allowing ourselves to experience the joy of health requires that we deal with relationships as clearly and concisely as possible in an effort to learn the lesson we have designed for ourselves. Each relationship will be focused on the balance of one particular aspect of self. Looking at the relationship to see if the lesson is focused in the physical, intellectual, or emotional aspect of self will help in our awareness and learning process. Family relationships will integrate lessons in all areas at different times. Relationships of the opposite sex, including marriage relationships in many instances, will have a primary focus. The primary focus for each individual will also vary with the period of the Law of Sevens we are experiencing. This is normal, as the focus in each period must be different as development occurs.

An example of this would be our first romantic love. Romantic love usually occurs in the third and fourth period of the Law of Sevens. Romantic love by nature has a physical focus. This physical focus is responsible for the term "myth of romantic love." The physical focus is not strong enough in romance to endure the experiences of time without the intellectual and Spiritual influences being present. We must grow through these learning periods of life, to balance and experience love from the focus of the intellectual and emotional aspects of self. Love must be of the body, mind and Spirit to endure in a relationship. This is essential for evolvement within our true state of energy balance.

If we are locked into the concept of romantic love, we are locked into the focus of the physical and we will not learn balance in this lifetime. Two Souls who marry for romantic love (physical focus) will find their marriage dissolving, unless both individual Souls are on the same path of unfoldment and attunement. One Soul cannot move forward to the development stage of intellectual focus or Spiritual focus if the other Soul is stuck in the physical focus, and have a marriage survive. This relationship will die from boredom, if nothing else. It is this type of relationship, where their friends will wonder "What do they do when they get out of bed?" You will hear comments of "What do they talk about?" This energy of boredom has spilled into the energy stream of their friends.

The same situation is true when a Soul is ready to focus on the emotional self instead of the physical self. If one Soul is focused on the emotional and another on the physical, they will suddenly find they have little in common. This relationship can erupt into violence and abuse, because it creates jealousy and anger. The ideal in marriage is to move along this path of growth together. When there is a true unconditional love that exists between two Souls this path is a path of commitment to the Dual Soul growth of both parties. It is understood on a Soul level by both Souls and is accepted as being the true and only love for that union of Souls. This is the ideal in a love relationship and marriage.

This is the ideal union for knowing the joy of health. It can give each Soul the freedom to seek balance. Emotional balance is hard for many Souls to reach in a solitary state; therefore, marriage has its assets in growth. The solitary state is the first lesson of relationships. Learning to give of ourselves to others is essential in forming lasting relationships. Emotional interaction must involve other Souls. The balance of body, mind and Spirit cannot be reached until each focus has been explored and understood by the Soul. Each focus is valuable in its place.

The important aspect is continued growth. Do not forget or refuse to change your focus in life. Resistance to change and resistance to relationships is a problem that we deal with daily. Relationships are equivalent to and are structured upon a foundation of communication. They are involved in a give and take, a flow of energy. This is true of all relationships, whether they are part of love, friendship, work or family. This energy sharing must be balanced and productive for the relationship to survive. Our relationships become our motivation to growth and living because they reflect an image of self. Resistance to relationships is a resistance to acknowledging self.

When a Soul finds itself fenced in by the belief system of the culture that creates a resistance to relationships, it will choose to leave Earth's plane and return with another life plan. The Soul has the freedom to abort the design and go for a more efficient one in another incarnation. When physical death appears to a Soul as the only way out of a life situation, it will choose the way of death and put that plan into action. Death occurs only by choice, but that choice is on a subconscious level.

Relationships that focus on emotional health are the path to Spiritual growth. Spiritual growth is true emotional health. On Earth it is easier and more acceptable to focus on the physical and intellectual paths. This can be done, with a focus toward health or disease in any of the three areas, as a Soul choice. In the integration of body, mind and Spirit each integral has the physical, intellectual and emotional function. Each is all and all is one, even in this concept. None can be separated, so speaking of one must include the total.

Look to your own life to evaluate your relationships. Each has its own complexity. For the sake of clarity in this explanation, we will focus on the male, female relationships of life. All relationships function within a similar framework so each can be understood from this explanation. We must look at relationships in terms of finding the lesson for us. Do not concern yourself with the lesson for the other party. It is not necessarily the same as yours and is not your concern.

Look honestly for reactions, do not look in judgment. Judgment does not belong in discernment. Judgment is, within itself, a negative force. There is no wrong. There is only the IS of life.

A Soul will, during the unfoldment of existence, first find romantic attractions of the opposite sex. These are physically focused attractions. The major thought in the mind is toward physical appearance (sex appeal), physical activities, physical creation, physical birth signs, physical work, and physical needs for support of our physical body. The physical focus is based on learning and belief systems of our physical world. It is controlled by our thinking mind, which early in life has only expanded to the physical sense response.

The mind and body always work in coordination whether it is a positive focus or a negative focus. As we progress through the Law of Sevens, we unfold. If we are lucky, we bloom like a beautiful rose, unfolding one petal at a time until we shine in full bloom. The physical focus is a material, commercial, physical need focus, which is the primary basis of our society. Many Souls live thousands of incarnations, trying to learn the lesson of physical resistance, existence, and material possessions.

The true lesson of physical focus is the preservation of our physical body to allow us the freedom to learn the lessons of the mind and Spirit. Any lesson of the physical can be integrated with the lessons of the mind and Spirit, without the physical focus being the primary focus. There is no right or wrong in the physical focus. There may be a resistance to the change of self that allows for growth of the mind and Spirit. This resistance is only another lesson and is not in itself right or wrong. It is simply the way of the Soul, in the process of learning.

As a Soul progresses through the Law of Sevens, it will shift from the physical into the mental and Spiritual focus as a natural process of unfoldment. This shift will act as a guide to the self, in evaluating the progress of unfoldment. This progress is essential to the process of growth. A Soul does not grow without change that is internal to self. Change will be manifested in our personality if not in the physical changes we may choose. During this period of unfoldment it is essential that we do not become obsessed with our own change. We need to change and unfold for the purpose of balance, not to define how great we think we are. Obsession with any facet of self creates imbalance.

This is why relationships are important in our life. Relationships will create exposure to other facets of self. For example, a man who loves his wife will choose to spend some time with her and this time will remove him from his normal intellectual pursuits. Business relationships will create an attachment to the physical world. They will afford exposure to contrary thoughts and practices. They will provide alternative paths and choices that must be made. They will challenge us to change in action to support change in beliefs. Without this challenge we would have a more difficult task of validation.

Validation of a change in beliefs occurs for us when we are willing to be known by those beliefs. Without relationships we can ascribe to a belief internally without the need to act on the belief in the physical world. Without the challenge to act on a belief change may never happen. In the presence of others, we would never know if we truly have the conviction of our new belief. We would continue to doubt self. Our belief system is the most difficult creation to change. It takes the courage of a well-founded new belief to support change in the eyes of friends and business associates. These are our relationships that we are looking to for validation of self.

True growth is allowing our fellow human to change without expressing judgment of that change, or judging the need for the change. When we can maintain the credibility of a relationship through the stress of unfoldment, it is a growing of two Souls rather than one. Those relationships that cannot understand the change of growth will dissolve from our world. This is as it should be. The drama that they created through the relationship has ended.

Each Soul will unfold at its own pace. The ability and depth of growth is an individual path. In this respect Souls of equal level will seek their own level for relationships. It is only at our own level or a greater level that relationships will continue to contribute to growth.

When a personal relationship has the proper balance of self from both parties, it will unfold at an enormous rate. The positive energy of one will expand the growth of the other and then the growth of energy of the partner will expand the partner's energy in turn. Their energies will flow in cycles with each other, allowing further and further expansion of growth. This creative growth pattern is the ideal in relationships and should be cherished.

This is a relationship that usually requires the closeness of marriage or family in our world, because of the continual interaction of the energy levels. Our society does not support communal living to the degree that would support such a relationship. It then must be found in the closeness of marriage. This balance in relationship is the master, consort role of relating and the roles themselves are interchangeable. The sharing is complete and comfortable. It is the oneness of self. It is the Father, Mother, and Spirit of us, integrated with the expansion of Spirit. This level of relationship allows each party to live the Ethical Values as a daily lifestyle.

The relationship of friends is the web of support that we create for self. These are the Souls of Spiritual memories that agree to be the mirror of self. On a physical level we will see people together that have the same interests in the physical world. These friendships happen because of our need to see ourselves in the reflection of friends. We are not comfortable with what we are not and have not grown into as part of our interests. This can be seen throughout our society. The people with identical belief systems gravitate to the Souls that are living that belief system. When we have a strong belief, we need friends with that same belief to feel "right" about ourselves. A friendship with someone that shares the same belief supports our belief and validates our wisdom. We will not be comfortable with or choose to spend time with Souls that are functioning within a different belief system.

Belief systems are the physical manifestation of a Soul's growth. Belief systems must change to allow growth. We will always seek our own level of growth. We will always experience change with growth, which will require a change of friends in our life unless the friends are experiencing the same growth path. When friends are on the same path, the friendship will survive throughout life. Many relationships of marriage and friendship have survived because of the refusal or resistance to change. These are Souls who are locked into a belief system. For these Souls this is where they must be. They are working with the lesson of resistance, which is the opposite of change.

Each lesson in life has its action and reaction. If we live a life of total resistance, we learn the value of openness which will become a later lesson for the Soul. When a Soul is learning the lesson of awareness and balance, it will move through these less advanced lessons with little if any difficulty. If we have learned the lesson previously, the experience will not appear as a reality in this life. It will be in this life physically, but the perception of importance will not be in us. We will live what we have learned and pay very little attention to the reaction of other people.

Many people will experience but fail to learn. Failure to learn is usually a failure to truly understand to the precise level of learning, which will require a re-experience in Earth life. When we leave Earth without learning our lessons, we will design the lesson into our next life plan. This is known in our world as Karma. Understand that Karma is not punishment; it is simply another class to graduate from at the end of our next life.

"Laundry" Day

Let us use a simple example to explain this. It is now "Laundry day" in your house. You gather everything together, throw it in the washer, change it to the dryer and presto, you have clean clothes. Now you go to your bedroom and you find another piece of dirty clothes. What are you going to do? Are you going to get upset and angry with yourself, scream and cry, curse and rave? Of course you aren't. You will drop the piece of forgotten clothing in the clothes hamper and it will be cleaned in the next wash. This is also a technique that we can use in our life situations.

This is how the Soul views Karma. It will be cleaned up on the next go around, so to speak. Karma is nothing for us to get excited about. That does not mean that we should avoid growth and do nothing. If that happens, we will spend many miserable years of living on Earth because of our lack of focus on developing awareness and understanding.

The relationships within families are all Soul relationships designed by Soul agreement. Many families come together by Soul design to work out or to help teach a Karmic lesson of great importance. This Karmic lesson may involve a family member, the world, a culture, a science or any combination of creations. The learning of that lesson or the manner in which it is worked out is not pre-determined. That part of the creation is an Earthly choice. The relationship is a Spiritual choice.

Frequently the choice is made with only one other member of the family with little or no Karma with other members. The level of involvement differs from Soul to Soul and may be with parents as well as other siblings and other relatives. The Karma may be the situational circumstance that makes the relationship experience important. When a Soul begins the design of his Spiritual prospectus of life, there are many issues that must be considered. Therefore, there will be many instances where family and circumstance are essential to the development of the prospectus. At other times, it may be the time in the development of Earth that creates the relationship.

There will always be important lessons to be learned within the family relationship that will impact on the overall growth of the Soul. Family relationships are never casual relationships from the standpoint of Soul evolution. The interaction of families is of the utmost importance in Soul development and should be valued. Despite the issues the Soul has chosen for his Earth life design, the relationship of the family will create choices to be made. Those choices help the Soul along the path of unfoldment. The family as a unit is the most supportive force for any Soul.

The family is not a mirror of self. It is a safety net of life. Family members have made a Spiritual commitment of unconditional love to each and every member of the family. This commitment is not a conscious commitment but a Spiritual commitment that is consistently in force on a super-conscious level. Despite the vicissitudes of living, that commitment will always be present. The symbolic expression of the family commitment was spoken of in the book we call the Bible, when the black sheep was welcomed home. In the family there is no judgment on a Soul level. There is only unconditional love.

Unconditional love is the true love of the Spirit. The love that we have for true friends, family, and partners in life has its source in the Soul memory for that Spirit that we know. Unconditional love does not judge. Unconditional love knows, accepts and supports the lessons of the Spirit self. It is the only true and lasting love that is available to our Spirit. Unconditional love is committed to the growth of the Dual Soul and Spirit Consciousness.

Unconditional love is a love of Soul memory. It can be recognized and practiced on a conscious level but the source of the love is from the core self. It is focused on the Spirit Consciousness rather than the physical self of Earth life. It is this Spirit focus of unconditional love that allows us to love our family, partner and friends without judging their physical reality. Physical action and reaction is not a reality of the Spiritual world. There is no judgment in the Spiritual world. There is no time. There is an abundance of love.

A Spiritual Soul will see all relationships with love. There will be no judgment. There will be no concept of time. The friend of many years will continue to be family today, despite the lack of contact within the physical realm. These Souls will continue a relationship on the Spiritual plane through the dream experience. This may not be a conscious awareness, but it is part of the Spiritual landscape for the Soul. Relationships can be viewed by all as the fiber of life. They provide the stage upon which the drama can be enacted. Without relationships we cannot and will not grow. Failure to validate relationships in life is a failure to validate self. Failure to develop relationships is a reaction to fear. Relationships are an action of love and support. We make our own choices in life, especially about relationships.

MARRIAGE

Marriage is symbolic of the need of each and every Soul to be married to Spirit. Marriage is the joining of the three persons within us – The Male (Father), The Child (Son) and the Mother (Holy Spirit). It is for the balance of this union that Earthly man in human form must marry of the opposite sex. Marriage of the opposite sex provides the balance of our Spiritual self. Without this balance we can only wish for the fruition of perfection in the eyes of Spirit, because we are not opening our human mind to understand both the male and female as equal. A good marriage, of awareness, understanding, and love, is a beauty to behold. The Souls of the partners shine, with the illumination of love as their internal reflection.

A marriage of love is as close to the perfect state as is possible for mortal humans on Earth. We are complete within but it is the external, physical self that seeks balance of the opposite sex. We are made totally in the image of Christ – We are as Christ is The Father, The Son, and The Holy Spirit. It was The Son that took human form; he is represented by the body. The Father is the Spirit (Mind and male symbol), the builder of all- for us the mind. The Holy Spirit is the Mother Spirit (heart and female symbol), the Spirit within us, the life force, the heart, the emotion of our Earthly presence. They are separate just as the Father, The Son, and The Holy Spirit are separate but the essence is one. The essence, or Spirit energy of self, cannot be separated.

Within each of us is all. But in human form our primary focus of any one lifetime will be indicated by what we aren't. Males are trying to learn to balance their female side and females are trying to learn to balance their male side. Marrying of the opposite sex helps with this balance and gives one the freedom to Be. This is evident in our world today, more than at any other time in the history of humankind. There many advanced Souls on Earth. These advanced Souls have a better balance of the male and female within. It is evident in their actions.

In some instances Soul development causes great moments of concern when a Soul of little advancement has a physical attraction to a Soul of great advancement. These relationships, when they end in marriage, cannot be tolerated happily for a lifetime by either party. The marriage that is motivated by physical need is the primary reason for the high divorce rate in our society. The evolution of the Earth is comparable to our human evolution. What happens within a world, a culture, a family, is the reaction to the thoughts and beliefs within our mind.

In the beginning of civilization our evolution was reflected in the evolution of the Earth as a direct result of our lifestyle, our knowledge and our understanding. This law has not changed. Today we create our world on a global, world, cultural, family, and individual basis, and it reflects precisely where our thinking mind is now.

The advanced Souls that are now on Earth have Soul memories of their effect upon the development of civilization. Those Souls learned and many are now at a stage of awareness where Soul memory is common. This is the history of evolution of both the human and Earth. New Souls, although they are entering a different atmosphere on Earth than the older Souls entered, do not have the experience of Soul evolution that older Souls have. They do not have the understanding, the learned lessons, the awareness of their Spirit Consciousness that an older Soul has learned, and they do not have the energy experience which is vital in our world today.

The joining together in marriage of a new Soul and old Soul cannot create the same depth of understanding and awareness within that two Souls of advanced evolution can produce. The new Souls are those that are "out there" today, without having learned many lessons, but they appear to be more visibly and actively in the process. This is the drama that is created because they are functioning essentially within the physical world. They have not yet discovered the inner world. These are the Souls that have no trouble going to war, of fighting on a daily basis, of being dishonest and judgmental. These are the Souls who are learning on a different level. There is no wrong in the way these Souls choose to learn. The learning process is essential and must include many dramas. All Souls follow the same Universal patterns.

Those old Souls who join in lessons do so out of the love they have for teaching. So even in seemingly perfect unions, the experience may dissolve the physical marriage, but the lesson is there and should be searched for carefully. Marriage is one of the best classrooms of our entire Earth school. Marriage can be even more of a helpful experience today, when the level of awareness is high and the couple enters marriage with the Soul memories of their past lessons together. They can, in this level of marriage, build more easily on the true characteristics of a Soul returning to Spirit. This, too, will take many incarnations.

There is a level in our evolution when our Soul memories are so profound that we stop incarnating to learn the lessons of early Soul evolution. This Soul will return to Earth to serve the masses and complete the Soul purpose of being in the image of Spirit. The lower level lessons of Earth life will trigger boredom in this Soul after a relatively short exposure in the physical world. The mundane activities and understandings of life will frustrate the vision of perfection that Soul dwells within.

We must work through our incarnations with progression from the physical into the Spiritual. Being locked into the physical lessons of Earth life for many incarnations will not produce progress. An aware Soul will remove itself from the experience in an effort to grow. Being in the religious life does not mean that an individual has reached the Spiritual. Religion is an occupation of man. That does not mean that it is Spiritual. Many times religion is greatly removed from the Spiritual and needs to be viewed in terms of a physical business rather than Spirit's business. Religion can be, for some Souls, a true avoidance of the physical world and its realities. That too presents an imbalance.

Many Souls choose to become involved in organized religion because of specific lessons they are seeking to learn. They may consider that they are married to Spirit. This marriage may suffer from the same problems that the physical Earthly marriages suffer. If one partner is at a different level of Soul evolution, the marriage is not a marriage of the Spirit. It is an interesting concept for us to believe that we are at the level of Soul development that we are on Earth to create. The belief and the choice create this search for the lesson of balance. No lesson is wrong. It simply is. As our choice, it will have its own impact on our Soul development.

The lesson of a marriage to Spirit will frequently have more to do with the lesson of human sexuality than reverence to the true Spirit. That is simply one of our lessons and one method of learning the lesson. For those who choose this path, it is their way. There are, in our world, many ways to learn to deal with human sexuality (identity). Another of the many ways is homosexuality.

Homosexual marriage is a reality in our world today. This too is an interesting way to deny the physical balance that was designed by Spirit. But each human act has its impact on growth. Of all the ways of marriage on Earth, the most efficient and final way is marriage of the opposite sex. This was the design of Spirit when Spirit made woman and man. That does not mean that in each and every incarnation marriage is a necessity. The lesson will determine the way of the path you choose. Progression will determine the need for balance in each of the trilocular levels of being.

As a Soul becomes more developed, it will not be acceptable to marry quickly simply for the sake of a mate. The desire for marriage will progress forward to the true concept of growth in partnership. This awareness will give Souls the freedom to be until the perfect partner in Soul development appears in one's life. It is better, from the standpoint of growth, for old Souls to progress alone rather than finding themselves constantly dealing with the lower level lessons of a less advanced partner. This will not be a major issue during the physical focus of development but it will become a crucial issue in the Spiritual focus of development.

The human need to search for a "Soul mate" is also destructive. In truth, Soul mates can be found everywhere in our life. They surround us. The true Spiritual partner could more accurately be defined as a twin Soul. Twin Souls are equal in their Soul evolution, will add more to our Soul growth, and be a more total partner in life than what our world knows as a Soul mate. Let us just say that the Spiritual generation gap can be very real for Soul mates despite chronological age. With twin Souls the chronological age, of this lifetime, has allowed for the awareness levels of each to have expanded into Soul memory. Without Soul memory there will be no recognition.

The most exalted purpose for marriage of two Souls is the presence of total unconditional love and sharing with a total commitment to Soul growth for yourself and your partner. Nothing else has the loftiness of true Soul purpose. This is the awareness of old Souls. New or less developed Souls are intensely directed towards physical attraction and infatuation. These Souls search for the drama of physical attraction. There will be emotional responses, jealousy, possessiveness, and fighting. The Soul consideration is not a reality of daily experience and will seldom be understood in the early marriages. In this too, there is a lesson. We must experience to learn. There is no other way.

The Earth culture today is more heavily populated with advanced Souls than it has ever been. This is universally reflected in awareness with parting in divorces as well as in all forms of marriage. Old Souls, desiring to incarnate, would not be comfortable or able to expand their growth, if they could not return to advanced Souls and enjoy sharing physically within Soul memory. This allows the Soul the freedom of retaining Soul memory just below or equal to consciousness from the beginning. It also gives the Soul the opportunity to begin with immediate Soul advancement. It makes living the lessons easier, more meaningful and more fun. It truly adds JOY to living.

Children should be viewed as old Souls, in a tiny physical form. Parents should see themselves as temporary custodians of those Souls, who have joined in the decision process of that Soul to incarnate. This joining is an acceptance of responsibility. The major responsibility is teaching this new little form how to thrive in the Earth's atmosphere again. The parent also has the responsibility of encouraging Soul memory while maintaining this small new being in lightness.

Many of life's lessons come to us in the form of physical lessons. With the advent of marriage and children, we create the responsibility for teaching. Teaching by example, as frequently as words, is our indication of the experience of the lesson for us. The concentration of this lesson for us, and the Soul that you are caring for through the physical years of growth, must be focused on health. It is from the focus of physical health that we survive in the physical body to the level of adult life. True health always searches for the balance of body, mind and Spirit. This is a Universal reality of childhood, adulthood, marriage, relationships, families or Soul development. Each facet of existence is within itself trilocular just as we are trilocular. We are a body, mind and Spirit that cannot be separated.

Our society can show with statistics that married men live longer than single men. This is accurate because of the improvement in eating habits and the decrease in the stress factors of searching. The joining of twin Souls will show an even greater increase in health because of the inner peace and joy they will share in addition to their Soul memory focus on physical health. Health is always health of body, mind and Spirit. But in the physical form the focus must start in the physical. There is no other way. Keeping the physical body healthy will release the energy for a healthy mind and Spirit.

Marriages that are based on verbal or physical abuse are not truly marriages under Spirit. They are two people, two Souls joining together for a space in physical time to learn a Karmic lesson. A Karmic lesson is a Soul lesson that has been tried before and resulted in failure. Karma is not punishment. It is a plan that we have designed for ourselves but have not yet been able to create. A plan that did not reach completion in another lifetime will be held over for completion in the next. Many times we will return as Souls to try again and again to learn the same lesson. We may try learning it with the same Soul of the past incarnation, but not necessarily.

If that lesson is a truly difficult experience, the two Souls involved in the process may decide to incarnate with other Souls who have learned that lesson and can approach it from a different perspective. This could be compared to the determination in physical life to learn to speak Spanish. If we chose to take Spanish in school three years in a row and still did not learn Spanish, we may decide to hire a tutor.

The final step in learning a lesson many times requires that Soul to incarnate to teach it to another Soul. Even in our society, the Soul memory knows that the only true way to learn is to teach. This understanding is a conscious Soul memory. And so it is on all planes. After working with the tutor and feeling that we know the lesson, we begin to teach it to others for the sake of repetition. It is the repetition that unlearns the old habits that kept us from learning the lesson in the first place. Therefore, the web of learning and teaching cannot be defined ever in singular terms because nothing is singular. Just as we are not singular even in physical form. Our lessons also are always easier when learned in partnership with another Soul, which gives them their own trilogy because of the everlasting presence of Spirit in our dramas.

Partnership of the opposite sex in marriage makes the cycle complete for those in human form. We are then a trilogy within and a trilogy without. We are, and our immediate environment is, comprised of The Father, The Son, and The Holy Spirit, because we are one, and we are separate. At that moment we manifest the ideal creation of all worlds. Partnership, a joining together, began with the beginning of time as Spirit's design in the concept of trilogy, in the separate state and in the state of Union. It is meant to maintain the Soul memory awareness of the union with Spirit. Spirit is also the Father, The Son, and The Holy Spirit. Spirit is Intellect (Universal knowledge), The Son (physical energy of man and Earth) and Heart (Mother Spirit-Spirit).

In human form, as the Son, we are Earth energy, a part of Nature. We are particles of energy fragmented from Spirit's energy. Our physical body is Earth energy and must be restored with Earth energy. The term Son on Earth is a derivation of the mystical or Spirit term of *Sun.* Son was given as a descriptive term to Jesus to denote the physical form of energy- the likeness of Spirit the Father. Jesus Christ was the Light, the Sun of Spirit. All humans are made in the Image of Spirit. We are the Light even without a conscious awareness of the Spirit within.

Any attempt, even by an advanced Soul, to explain the vastness and complexity of Spirit, the Father and the concept of creation, is impossible except to value the utmost in simplicity for it is indeed simple in its complexity. The need for an explanation of the creation is apparent but that in itself is another book. For now we will offer that which seems necessary to clarify the concept of us on Earth and our relationship to Earth.

An aware Soul will understand every explanation and the unaware will argue every word. That too is as it must be. Understanding can be used as a guideline of our own individual awareness. If we don't at first understand, have faith in knowing that additional readings will raise our awareness level. The understanding is in the essence of truth, which is an unconscious understanding for us in the process of reading. Many explanations have been presented to the world in an attempt to reach more Souls. They are in essence all one. Essence is in our terms "energy." The energy of the truth of the explanation is the same. The presentation is given as is appropriate to the writing and the Soul energy towards which the writing is focused.

A marriage of two Souls, on the same path under Spirit, is the perfect union to remind us of the perfect union. These perfect unions come in the latter stages of Soul development primarily. They should be honored as a gift of awareness of the Soul. At times there may be a Soul who chooses to join with a younger fragment Soul of its own to teach. This would be done in an effort to raise all fragments of the Soul to the same level. Souls and their fragments must come together as one Soul to return to the Soul of Spirit, in unity. In this instance, marriage would be a perfect union. Souls that are from the same family of Souls are on the same energy vibrations and will have an intense interest in the soul growth of the marriage partner. This is the true twin Soul for any lifetime.

In our Book of "God," the partnership of the male and female in marriage was again the union for balance.

As our human Soul evolves, the relationship of man and woman is becoming more truly the partnership that Spirit designed it to be on Earth. Throughout Earth time the relationship of the male and female in the marriage partnership has many times failed as a partnership, although it may have sustained as an Earth marriage.

Understanding that our growth depends upon balancing the body, mind and Spirit makes it easier to grasp an awareness of the true need of equality in marriage. In equality a balance of the male and female will develop within each partner. Neither party will find themselves stuck in a role. There should be no roles. There should be a sharing in equality for total growth and awareness of the Soul. Man and woman were created equal, to live equally, to learn equally and to participate in marriage equally. Each partner has the same virtues but in different balance. The marriage of man and woman allows each to be whole and in balance.

The concept of parenting within Spirit's union is the joy, happiness and health of aware Souls on a mission of faith. There is trust and a knowingness in the child as well as the parents. This presents marriages with glory, wisdom and knowledge. It is another experience in the unity of us. The ideal time for parenting within our society, at the present time, is in the fourth and fifth period of the Law of Sevens. In the space and time that our society will next enter, this period may be extended for the fourth, fifth and sixth periods of the Law of Sevens. It is not yet time for a perfect extension to that period. As the awareness of health grows, parenting in later life will become a physical reality in our world without the problem of physical complications. At present, the physical complication of the infant may be secondary to the physical health of both parents. When we reach this period in our society the energy drain on our cellular structure, due to eating improperly and negative thinking, can be harmful to the development of a perfect human energy form. The Souls who choose to enter this imperfect physical body do so for their own Soul lesson. This joint decision between parents and child fulfills the needs of all. There are no accidents. Awareness can erase the need for this lesson for many advanced Souls in the continuation of their Soul development.

For those in marriage, know thyself and thy partner. Cherish, love and share in Spirit's union of grace. Look to each other for a commitment to the growth of the Soul. Health of the physical is the place to begin. The energy released will help open the mind and the Spirit. As the body, mind and Spirit become balanced, the life you share together will be one of true equality and growth. It will be filled with love, joy and happiness. Your cup will runneth over! Contribute to each other in all facets of growth.

All marriages should be a "coming home" for the Soul. If the marriage begins with a physical focus, that is a marriage of that level of development. If the love between the partners is the unconditional love of the Spirit then the commitment will be there for growth and development in both. Change and growth will be necessary for both Souls or resistance will be necessary for both Souls, if the marriage is to survive on the physical plane of Earth. Marriage is a unity of self and our partner. Separation cannot productively occur on any level and have the marriage endure. Within unity is total freedom of self. Freedom of self does not depreciate the concept of unity by separation of the physical, but expands it into the freedom of growth.

We will subconsciously commit separation by developing other interests in life to focus upon. This is a denial of unity as it is a denial of self. It is destructive to the concept of marriage. This is an unconscious resistance to the natural growth through unity of Souls. This Soul is denying and resisting change within. If there is no growth and joy in a union, change is an alternative, a choice for us. Change should be faced with our love for growth, rather than our fear of change.

Consciously, we should marry for growth just as we live for growth. We should be open to growth within a marriage rather than seeking change outside the marriage. Perspectives of the marriage can be changed, if both people are willing to look within for cause rather than to look without for blame.

The mirror of self can become frightening for a Soul to encounter, and this will create resistance within the partner when growth is singular. The mirror of self can serve to inspire the Soul within, if understanding is there. When we seek the energy of a marriage partner the energy traits of self will be visible within the energy traits of the partner. It is easier to discern features within another than within the self. Grow from the experience, because that was the basis for seeking the experience.

The ideal in marriage is that perfect band of positive energy that inspires the growth, one from the other. The centripetal force of that positive energy pulls the partners of the marriage tighter and tighter into the energy band of awareness and understanding of self and the unity of being. The gold band of the wedding ring is symbolic of that gold band of Spiritual energy which unites a man and woman in marriage. Development of that band of Spiritual energy will allow for expanded Soul growth, within the Spiritual unity of marriage.

We develop our Soul in the state of unity, with Spirit and with a partner. Spirit in her creative wisdom made us a trilogy of self, just in case there is no "coming home" on Earth. It is still a reality that the positive force of energy expands with the addition of another positive force. Therefore marriage is an ideal experience of Earthly life to promote and expand the growth of the Soul.

Marriage

A marriage of man and woman, committed to growth within the unity of that marriage, is a marriage under the positive and creative force of Spirit. A good marriage creates a Trinity upon Earth.

Metaphysical Teachings

Seven Levels of our invisible energy

BEING

A state of being (life) that we create from the beliefs and behaviors of our dual soul mind and emotions.

GOD

Accepting the Good within us as our Christ Consciousness and the essence of our eternal Spirit.

TRUTH

The absolute consistency of our inspired thoughts, communication, and our physical behavior.

KNOWLEDGE

The absolute truth of understanding ourselves in relationship to God, Nature, and all of humanity.

ENERGY

The dynamic force of light within us that is created by electricity and magnetism becoming one.

CREATION

The fractal pattern of life that unifies our electromagnetic energy with physical matter.

HUMAN and DIVINE Relationships

The energy interaction of our physical nature and our Divine Nature both internally and externally.

THE SPIRIT SELF

The question of us and our relationship to Spirit has been debated since the beginning of time. There are those who feel that we should not refer to ourselves as being of Spirit. There are those who feel that we are our own Spirit. There are those who feel that there is no Spirit. There are those who feel that we are only physical matter. There are those that see Spirit as a formidable force who will punish us in hell and damnation. For every person, there is a separate belief that lives inside the self.

What is right and what is wrong should not be a question that concerns us. Spirit is. Spirit is an image. Spirit is all that is. Spirit is energy. Spirit is life. Spirit is Spirit. Without Spirit, we would not be and live as energy beings.

Belief in that which cannot be seen is difficult for some Souls after they enter the plane of Earth. Their concepts of reality are focused on that which is physical. They do not have an awareness of self that searches deeper into the Soul, into the very Spirit of us. Attachment to the physical concept does not mean that they are wrong. They are, more accurately, unaware. Our lack of awareness does not change what is. The growth of the Soul is many times reflected in the level of awareness, but this will not always be a conscious awareness.

Nevertheless, awareness will be there at the core level and it can be detected by other advanced Souls. Soul memory becomes overshadowed with the realities of the physical universe for that individual. Association with an advanced Soul will trigger the awareness in a Soul that is sleeping.

When we speak of Spirit or All That Is, we are speaking of an internal sense. We are speaking of love. We are speaking of the inherent traits of Spirit that are mirrored within our Soul. We are speaking of the Good within us. We are speaking of the Spirit self. Each person holds within some Good – or some Spirit. Spirit is good and Good is Spirit essentially. When we deny Spirit we deny the Good within us. When we deny Good we deny the Spirit within us. The traits of Spirit cannot be learned because they are inherent within each of us. They need only to be acknowledged and used to be our Birthright.

Love, truth, and perfection are the image of Spirit that is within each of us. They must be acknowledged and used for us to appear as Spirit on Earth. Mirroring the image of Spirit as a human being makes us a more perfect Son of Spirit on Earth. Spirit does not require that we view Spirit as supernatural. Spirit is Man, and Man is Spirit. There is no separation between the two. The Spirit state is the ultimate Soul evolvement for us.

In us, Spirit is manifested as the Good, the Spirit of Life, the Soul. These do not exist outside of us but must be within as part of our everyday life, part of our

Being. We cannot say one thing and do another. If we do we are speaking not with the voice of the Spirit within, but with the voice of the physical self, the ego that is the control function for us.

When we were created we were created from the energy essence of Spirit. We are the Son of Spirit, created from a seed of energy of the Spirit. In our world our sons are created from our seeds, in the same Spirit concept that the energy from self creates another self. Remember, how proud each new father is of his child, Spirit is also proud of us. We are Spirit's children. Each birth recreates us, in the eyes of Spirit. And in each of us is that energy essence of All That Is. In each person is the Spirit self. In each person is the genetic energy of Spirit, the Spirit of us. At birth each child is love, truth and perfection.

Awareness of this birthright is our challenge. This cannot be a superficially learned, intellectual awareness. It must be a Soul awareness that integrates our body, mind and Spirit. We are eternally seeking balance of the physical, mental, and Spiritual awareness within. Spirit placed us on Earth in a physical presence. The physical lesson is the first lesson of the Soul. We must learn to be balanced in the physical body, before we can function totally in the mental and Spiritual realm of self. Balance is sought through multiple Earth incarnations, in our effort to balance the body, mind and Spirit on the physical plane. An unbalanced Spirit would create a Spiritual chaos in the Spiritual planes. High level Spirits have learned the lesson of physical balance. When we find people in our world creating chaos on a physical level, they have not found balance within their physical sense.

In the physical realm, we have complete and total access to the Universal knowledge and to the Spirit of Spirit. We have the totality of mind and Spirit. We have the reality of Earth and our physical self. We have everything available within the Universe for complete and perfect balance of self. We have only the challenge to develop our awareness of the need for balance to be complete. When we understand and integrate self, we will be conscious of the Spiritual levels of consciousness and we will have an acute awareness of the physical and mental levels of consciousness. This is not an aberration of the physical self. We all have multiple senses that we do not use because of our resistance to changing our belief system.

If we did not believe that planes could fly, we could not have invented the airplane. If we did not believe that we could live on the ocean floor, we would not have invented the submarine that allows us to be on the ocean floor. If we did not believe that we could take a spaceship to the moon, we could not have accomplished this feat. If we do not believe that we have senses other than the five physical senses that we use, we will not attempt to understand or use our other senses. It is our belief system that restricts us.

This challenge is presented to us daily in the form of Earth lessons. Nothing in Earth life is an accident. The most insignificant appearing instances of our life are of value in the balance we are seeking. If we believe that everything that happens to us is circumstantial, we will not understand the lesson that is within the incident. It is with the happenings of our life that we build our awareness. The building itself we have planned, not in a predetermined concept but in the concept of goal orientation. For each plan that we have developed, we have created several paths to follow to reach the same goal. The path that we take in life becomes our choice. We know on an unconscious level where we want to go, but our choice on the conscious level will determine how we get there. The concept of lessons is difficult for some of us to understand or accept. But in the reality of our physical world, our life is our classroom. Living is our lesson.

When we are a student we attend school each day. We must go to a specific classroom to learn a specific lesson. In each hour of our day, our class is different and our lesson is different. At the end of our educational study program, we will have learned to combine all of the knowledge that we have gained into an intellectual concept of whatever specific we have been studying. We will have learned to take all of this valuable information, and balance it together to make ourselves aware of how we can best function in our chosen field of endeavor.

When we start this balancing process, we will not be using only the information that we learned in the classroom of our school. This learned information will be perceived in relationship to the life knowledge and belief systems that we have absorbed from the moment of birth. We will be balancing every influence of our life. We will discard some beliefs, some learning, and we will attach ourselves more firmly to others. This is the constant flow of consciousness energy that is designed to help us seek the balance of awareness. This is the lesson of Earth existence. Life is a river constantly flowing, constantly changing, constantly seeking that calm pool where there is peace and where there is balance.

Our lessons of life are a mirror repetition of our classroom lessons. We learn by what we do, think, see, hear, sense, feel, smell, touch, taste and know. We, as human beings, are an integration of experience of body, mind, and Spirit. This is not one experience but it is the totality of experience within the space of all Earth sojourns as well as the experience of existence on other planes. We have always been fascinated with the study of self. We have dissected, examined, explored and believed that we understand our physical, mental and Spiritual realities. Truly this is an illusion.

We should spend time studying Nature and we will understand ourselves. In all of Spirit's Creation there is consistent trilocular duplication. Nothing is new. Everything is designed in the image of Spirit. The Father, The

Son, and The Holy Spirit. Everything and all of man is love, truth, and perfection. Everything in Nature is designed in an intricate cellular formation of balance, from the minute cell to the reality of its completion in physical form. So, too, are we. Everything exists within its own rhythm of balance. So, too, do we as human beings. We are only another creation of Nature by Spirit. We are one with the Earth. We are of the Earth.

In our study of self we have frequently concentrated on one component part, to the exclusion of all other parts. It is not only a physical world, an intellectual world or a Spiritual world. One cannot exist without the other. We are an integrated being. We are separate units, but we are one self. We are an intricate balance that is natural to the core self but unnatural to our conscious awareness. The Earth lesson is awareness of this balance. Life is the balanced integrated participation of all of self. Life is showing appreciation for the physical, the intellectual and the Spiritual person that we are. No one part of us can be in the majority. The Soul purpose is learning how to totally integrate the equal parts for complete balance. It is in finding this balance that we reach perfect health. If we were only physical, we would be the soil of Earth. If we were only mind, we would be an element of energy floating in space without direction. If we were only Spirit, we would be an element of energy with direction.

We are Spirit and we have direction. We can capture and integrate the energy of knowledge. We can personally perform physical action. We can direct our minds and Spirit through the physical body. We have the power of integration. Assuming the image of the physical is a choice of the Spirit. Many times in our Soul experience, we use a physical body in the physical sense, rather than in the integrated sense of Spirit as the whole of us, as I am now doing. With Soul evolution into the integrated state of awareness and understanding, it becomes more difficult for the Soul to remain within the physical body.

For us to be functional on Earth, we must be an integration of all three parts of the Trilocular Self. It is the Spirit Self, our Spirit that provides the direction in being. Direction can be defined here as Will and Intent. The Spirit must integrate with the mind for the knowledge, the intellectual concepts. The mind then integrates with the body to perform the physical action.

The direction of the Spirit is always positive and always enlightening. There is no negative influence within the Spirit. When we do not hear our Spirit but follow the direction of our ego, we can live in negative energy. This ego energy causes the problems that are prevalent within our world. Our awareness must wait for a more perfect balance to be achieved, before the human state can be understood. Not hearing and not understanding the Spirit

Self is not understanding the true direction of our own physical life and what it is attempting to teach us.

Good is as good does. We prove our own validity as a "son of Spirit" in our actions. The Spirit Self is not directed by the physical self. The Spirit Self is directed in the ways of our eternal energy or All That Is. The Spirit Self is: Love Spirit, thyself and thy neighbor as thyself, which can be said to love everyone equally. When we learn to create Good in relationship to All, we will have learned to follow the direction of our Spirit. We will be following the path of awareness. We will have truly integrated the Spirit self or eternal energy into our physical life.

Look within. Goodness is not a concept that can be grasped from the air. Goodness is truth. Truth is the Spirit in action. Truth is a living Spirit. Truth is the validity of life. Truth is Spirit within us. An illusion of goodness, of truth, is a product of verbal creation that has no Spiritual validity. It has no reality of reaction or credibility within the physical world. It is an illusion that exists in the mind of one who lives in fear of self. Looking within is the perfect path to balance. We cannot look to others to show us our illusions, because in looking externally we are creating new illusions. Nothing in our reality exists "out there," within the reality of another person. We cannot blame our mother, our father, our spouse, or our friend. We are responsible for our own agenda in life. We created the goal and we have made our choices. We have created our own illusions. We have created ourselves and our physical world. It is at this point of looking within, that we suddenly stop and say, "I am not responsible for ____________." Indeed, we are!

Accepting personal responsibility for self is a difficult concept for most people. It is always more comfortable to blame another than to look internally at ourselves. Blaming avoids the issue of looking within. Blaming totally avoids the lesson that we are trying to learn. It avoids the recognition of truth. It denies our eternal energy. It creates a new illusion for the ego. It is comfortable for the physical self. Each Soul is here to learn his own individual lessons. We are attracted to situations that will help us learn those lessons. There will be other Souls involved who are there to help us with our lesson. In helping us they will be working on their own lesson. It will not be the same lesson.

Because the lessons are not the same, it is essential that we look within. No one is responsible for the lesson of the other participants. We are responsible for ourselves and our own personal growth. We are responsible for nothing else. Any individual that attempts to learn through the veil of an "I know it all" belief will learn very little, and perhaps nothing.

Personal growth occurs only within the vibrations of positive energy. Growth and negative energy are opposing forces so they cannot create within a mind.

Negative energy forces are the Universal reason for creating change in the drama of life. As we abuse ourselves and other people, our Universal lesson of love becomes dramatically important and essential to our growth and change. No one else can ever grow and change for us. Our growth and change are always our personal responsibility.

Accepting the responsibility for the actions of self, looking at those actions to determine the truth for us, can be physically uncomfortable. But without looking within, there will never be balance. Without learning the lesson, we cannot expect promotion to the next class. Life is like the classrooms of our physical world. If we can't master reading and writing, we may never reach arithmetic. It is the Law of Physical Balance. We cannot proceed to take the next step forward, until we balance the step that we are in. If we attempt to move ahead of ourselves, we will not be living truth.

It is within the truth of self that we find the Spirit Self – the Spirit of Being. Within the Spirit of Being is the Joy of Health – the balance of self that we are eternally seeking on Earth. Seek your Joy with the awareness of the openness of your Soul memories. Seek your joy of life by living and using the love, truth and perfection of your Spirit Self. When we seek enlightenment the light will be found within. Joy is love. Love must begin by loving yourself. Live your entire life, in all of its many aspects, in peace and joy towards yourself and with other people.

Trinities of Ethical Values

Love Truth Equality

Independence Freedom Personal Responsibility

Integrity Strength Courage

Patience Understanding Support

Unity Commitment Integration

Faith Trust Humility

Honor Value Respect

Organization Form Structure

Discipline Knowledge Passion

Free Will Free Choice Free Intention

Compassion Cooperation Communication

Kathy Oddenino Books

Bridges of Consciousness: *Self Discovery in the New Age*

$14.95 – ISBN 0-923081-01-1

Sharing: *Self Discovery in Relationships*

$14.95 – ISBN 0-923081-02x

Love, Truth & Perception: *A Spiritual and Philosophic View of Human Destiny*

$14.95 – ISBN 0-923081-03-8

Healing Ourself: *Growing Beyond the True Cause of Disease*

$24.95 – ISBN 0-923081-04-6

Depression: *Our Normal Transitional Emotions*

$24.95 – ISBN 0-923081-05-4

The Journey Home: *Our Evolving Consciousness*

$33.00 – ISBN 0-923081-0

Spirit Consciousness: *Our Intelligent Design*

$29.95 – ISBN 978-0-923081-07-2

www.kathyoddenino.com

www.ingramcontent.com/pod-product-compliance
Lightning Source LLC
Chambersburg PA
CBHW020600270326
41927CB00005B/112